BOUNDLESS CURES

An Insider's Guide to Natural Healing in the New Millennium

Marc S. Micozzi, M.D., Ph.D.

Table of Co

Table of Contents (continued)

Introduction

Humans possess an innate self-healing potential, an "inner wisdom of the body." Accessing this self-healing system is the primary goal of the healing arts. And addressing the cause of any illness is the first step towards accessing the body's own healing potential. However, modern medicine's primary focus is on suppressing symptoms instead. The problem is, suppressing symptoms with pharmaceutical drugs can compromise and diminish the body's natural ability to heal itself. Which is why natural, nonpharmaceutical measures should generally be the first approach—not the last resort. Unfortunately, far too many promising natural therapies—and cures—have been derailed for the sake of profit and political gain. But in the following chapters, I'll tell you how you can find these effective treatments—and put them to use for you and your loved ones starting today.

Always on the side of science,

Marc S. Micozzi, M.D., Ph.D.

CANCER ANSWERS FROM A TRUE INSIDER

Part 1: Cancer Answers from a true insiderr

Chapter 1

The "ONE WORD" battle plan
to crushing cancer

Until this very moment in medical history, the common notion in the mainstream crusade against cancer is: *Chemo is as good as it gets.*

Of course, I've always known this was untrue. And if you've been curious enough to poke your head up from the sea of cancer misinformation we're drowning in, maybe you've glimpsed the truth for yourself.

Chemotherapy is a desperate grasping at straws in an effort to "kill the cancer before we kill the patient." But it also blatantly ignores the mountains of complementary medical research proving that cancer can be prevented and treated without this.

But in the last few years, even some of the most die-hard mainstreamers have taken notice of a new form of cancer treatment called anti-angiogenesis. It's radically different from the "poison and pray" chemo approach to treatment. An approach many of us have had to watch loved ones suffer through. But as you'll see, the difference in methodology is only the first of many reasons to have hope.

The "AH-HA!" moment
modern medicine was praying for

In 1998, *The New York Times* created a media frenzy…they reported a scientist by the name of Dr. Judah Folkman had discovered a way to eradicate tumors in mice. The frenzy swelled to such heights that Nobel laureate, Dr. James Watson was quoted as saying, "Judah is going to cure cancer in two years." And, in effect, he did. So why haven't you heard about it over the past decade?

Indeed, Dr. Folkman was a special kind of scientist. I admired his natural instincts in following the science so much, in fact, that even before the media frenzy in 1998, I personally invited him to speak in Philadelphia to a standing-room only crowd of distinguished physicians and scientists. (This was when I was director of The College of Physicians of Philadelphia, and I was honored to have him come and enlighten my guests).

At that point, Dr. Folkman had already been following this particular scientific revelation for over 30 years.

It all started with the question…how can tumors grow so fast and so aggressively?

During his time at the National Naval Medical Center in Bethesda, MD, he had noticed cancer cells were unable to organize into tumors bigger than a few millimeters *in vitro* (meaning in test tubes, outside of the body). So somehow tumors were dependent upon the human body for growth.

And then he saw it.

Your body is being hijacked

Dr. Folkman was already considered to be the founder of angiogenesis research, so he knew what to look for. But what exactly is angiogenesis?

It's your ability to grow new capillary blood vessels in the body.[1] It's a special process. And in balance, it shouldn't happen too often (mostly during menstruation for women, wound healing, and of course, while a fetus is still within the womb).

But when the body needs to divert more blood and nutrients to a specific area, it activates endothelial cells in the lining of blood vessels to release enzymes called proteases. These allow endothelial cells to "bust out" of the current capillary they're in and form new capillaries. This ability to form new blood vessels obviously helps with the healing process, human growth, and supplying much-needed nutrition throughout your body.

But it can turn deadly...

The big break came when Dr. Folkman applied his knowledge of angiogenesis to cancer research. For decades, researchers had marveled at a tumor's ability to grow exponentially larger in such a short amount of time. But what if these cancerous tumors were *using* your body to feed themselves and even spread elsewhere?

It wasn't long after that Dr. Folkman proved tumors secrete angiogenesis-inducing factors (mitogens) which cause neighboring normal capillaries to extend and supply blood to the tumor.[2]

It was an incredible step—one that could eventually lead us away from the "poison and pray" treatment of chemotherapy, which oncologists appear so eager to administer these days.

This single hypothesis spawned nearly uninterrupted breakthroughs for almost 40 years. It's the kind of watershed moment about which every scientist dreams. Two of the biggest breakthroughs came in identifying a whole family of angiogenic peptides[3] and in showing that once you shut them down, you can choke tumors out of existence.[4]

What does that mean for you and your family?

"Angiogenesis research will probably change the face of medicine in the next decades, with more than 500 million people worldwide predicted to benefit from pro- or anti-angiogenesis treatments"[5]

That is a quote from the January 2006 issue of *Nature*—and they're right.

Anti-angiogenesis therapy is already turning heads in research facilities and hospitals all over the world. That's why over $4 billion has recently been spent researching anti-angiogenesis, making it one of the biggest medical research initiatives in history.[6]

In fact, there are already 374 clinical trials in the works and vested interests are practically drooling over the profit potential.[7]

Sadly, Dr. Judah Folkman passed away recently at the age of 75, but the research he started is now finally thriving. New angiogenesis inhibitors are being discovered all the time. Doctors are now witnessing tumors shrink and in some cases wither away completely. In fact, this therapy should be able to make chemotherapy extinct someday.

But the best news is that you don't have to wait another minute to start putting this revolutionary technique to work for yourself. As usual…

Nature is already seventy steps ahead of us

…And counting. The great news for all of us is that these angiogenesis revelations have shone light on an entire world of natural anti-angiogenesis compounds.

Much in the same way you might support your immune system with vitamin C, or your joints with Boswellia or your prostate health with saw palmetto…there are safe and natural ways to support your body's angiogenesis balance.

I'll reveal some of nature's most powerful—and readily available—anti-angiogenesis treatments in chapter 3. But first, a closer look at one of the most powerful cancer cures ever discovered—and the insidious story of how it was derailed by the very people in charge of "protecting" our health.

Chapter 2

The natural cancer secret: vitamin C

The proven cancer revelation—
pushed aside for profits!

In 1984, a senior staff scientist for the National Cancer Institute (NCI) and a personal friend of mine was on the verge of a medical epiphany. She had gathered towering piles of PROVEN research regarding a downright *ordinary* substance. Vitamin C.

She was a part of the "crash program" to uncover as much as we could on the relationship between diet, nutrients, and cancer. And had taken it upon herself to gather and review a decade's worth of small, very sound studies on vitamin C. And what she found was staggering.

In fact, this tireless researcher reviewed over 46 separate epidemiological studies. She found that 33 of them revealed vitamin C offered **significant protection against cancer...particularly for esophageal, pancreatic, stomach, lung, and breast cancers.**[8]

Thirty-three out of 46. That's a 71% rate of positive results!

And in subsequent studies, vitamin C continues to produce jaw-dropping results...

- One study in mice showed vitamin C could rob a tumor of its power source—literally halting any new growth.[9]

- In the prominent medical journal *Prostate*, it was reported to be a "potent anticancer agent for prostate cancer cells."[10]

- It was shown to be a CRITICAL element in your body's ability to resist neoplasia—the formation of abnormal cells.[11]

Research had even been performed by two-time Nobel laureate, Linus Pauling leading him to controversially proclaim, "This substance can prevent cancer."

Imagine. A real cancer breakthrough sitting right under the nose of the NCI the whole time. And all they had to do was look beyond the cutting, burning, and poisoning. To consider safer, natural approaches. And they didn't even have to look far. This secret weapon was found just starting with the basics! Of all things, vitamin C.

And yet, tragically, chances are you still haven't heard the potential of vitamin C for the prevention and treatment of cancer.

There was one BIG PROBLEM...

When this dedicated researcher finished her work, she went proudly before our political bosses to deliver the revolutionary news. Was she congratulated? Was she asked to present her findings to an expanded panel of her superiors? *Was she even listened to?*

No. The National Institutes of Health (NIH), the guardian of this nation's health and wellbeing, wasn't interested in her findings. They weren't interested in the success rates, shrinking tumors, or how amazingly simple, affordable, and effective her discovery was.

I know it sounds unbelievable. We're talking about a senior scientist, with a stack of credible research in hand. The sheer weight and height of which she actually carried into her superior's office to try to convey the potential in person.

But the sad truth is...the NIH already *had* a "natural cancer plan." And vitamin C didn't fall in line. The "science bureaucrats" ignored a hard-working, dedicated scientist with more-than-promising results in hand. All because they had already invested themselves in a plan that would just be too hard to stop.

What was so good that they could afford to ignore this colleagues' staggering scientific findings?

Beta-carotene. Those two words (and tens of millions of dollars) single-handedly derailed this nation's entire medical establishment—for decades—from finding a PROVEN cure for cancer. Because in 1984, a monumental initiative was mandated. The goal was to make beta-carotene the *cancer treatment darling* for the upcoming century.

One study is all it took to get the NIH frothing at the possibilities. Just one study, compared to the stack of research my colleague uncovered on vitamin C. You see, beta-carotene is a plant-derived form of vitamin A. And in 1981, an influential English scientist (who had studied in Nazi Germany during their earlier war on cancer) in an influential English scientific journal, simply asked a simple question based on a study showing the higher one's vitamin A levels; the less likely they were to develop lung cancer. You see, beta-carotene was of interest because it's a water-soluble, plant form, that can be converted in humans to Vitamin A, which is fat-soluble (and therefore potentially toxic). So, NCI was really looking for Vitamin A activity thru giving "safe' beta-carotene. Of course, we now know that even that thinking was faulty. Many people do not convert beta-carotene to Vitamin A at all, or only a little, or only under certain conditions. SO, beta-carotene can not be considered a reliable source of Vitamin A from plants. So, the NCI immediately jumped to all the wrong conclusions.[12]

And conveniently for the NIH, there was a synthetic form of beta-carotene already on the market. Readily available for testing. So they jumped right in. (Though it's likely that's not the only reason, which I'll explain in just a minute.)

Flash forward two years and the NIH had issued a large-scale clinical trial. (The cost of which soared into the tens of millions.) And word had spread to the press that "beta-carotene would save us all from cancer!"

All the while, several colleagues from the USDA Human Nutrition Research Center and I were uncovering evidence of the exact opposite.

We actually looked to the past and reviewed a dozen smaller studies on beta-carotene. And we found no correlation between blood levels of beta-carotene and cancer. We also looked at over 30 studies following the results of the British Empire Cancer Campaign. We looked at the foods that consistently showed protective effects against cancer. Then we used the latest, state-of-the-art technology to identify the carotenoid content of each of these foods. And they were *not* high in beta-carotene. But they *were* high in vitamin C and other nutrients.

There was essentially no reason for the NCI to "bet" on beta-carotene. No reason to proceed with multi-million dollar, taxpayer-funded clinical trials that gave synthetic beta-carotene to people already at increased risk for cancer.

But it was too late. The NIH had already let word leak out to the media about their new "darling." And seemingly overnight, thousands of everyday citizens were taking beta-carotene for cancer. All before a full-scale clinical trial had even started!

In fact, once the clinical trial got underway, it was hard to organize the control group of patients *because so many people were already taking beta-carotene*. In the medical science world—that's counting your eggs long before you even have the chicken...

But why, oh why was the NIH throwing caution (and a proven cure!) to the wind?

Because the reward was just too great. And unfortunately, I'm not talking about saving lives. When it comes to questionable judgments taking place in our more *"infallible"* institutions—always look at the advisory board.

In this particular case—a member of one of the *National Cancer Institute's* advisory boards happened to be a senior science officer at the manufacturer of a leading synthetic beta-carotene available at the time. And there it is. The shameful dots should be easy enough to connect. If beta-carotene became the "chosen one" amongst the NIH, record profits were *guaranteed. Even before results were ever gathered, and regardless of what the results showed.*

All the while, sealing the fate of a TRUE CANCER ANSWER to sit on the shelf, collect dust, and be kept from you.

One day I asked another scientist how the NCI could continue to ignore all the evidence about vitamin C. He explained that two-time Nobel Prize winner Linus Pauling had given vitamin C a "bad name." In the government's eyes, he was too vocal about its benefits. And the NCI couldn't afford to be seen as "kooky" or "fringy." Better to be just plain wrong. Meanwhile, Linus Pauling single-handedly held as many Nobel Prizes as the entire scientific bureaucracy of NIH put together. But the NCI prefers to be "often wrong, but never in doubt."

In fact…

We discovered many things when we began to do research with the USDA. First, we found that the nutritional quality of foods had declined drastically each decade during the 20th century right through the 1980's.

Second, almost all the healthy foods that are known to prevent cancer in fact are not high in beta-carotene. But we did find that these foods *are* high in vitamin C and a lot of other carotenoids that no one had heard of before, including **lutein, lycopene,** and **beta-cryptoxanthine.**[13] All powerful nutrients that you can easily stock up on through the green, leafy vegetables you get at the grocery store.

And all the NCI managed to prove, tens of millions of dollars later, was that beta-carotene did *not* prevent cancer. And that, in fact, **cancer could actually increase by over 25% in some when using the synthetic, isolated beta-carotene of our friendly drug company.**[14]

And all along, this flawed approach of the NCI—using the wrong doses, forms, and isolated synthetic nutrients—led to mixed results. Which of course opened the door to criticism by pharmaceutical-led mainstream medical science and oncology. Who continue to argue that nutrition won't work against cancer.

I even went so far as to formally predict the failure of this flawed approach. I knew it wouldn't work thanks to my work with the USDA, who actually knew something about nutrition. So I wrote up a scientific paper using the flawed and ill-fated example of beta-carotene. But my paper got caught up by my "political" bosses at the NCI…protecting their cancer empire, covering up their ignorance of human nutrition, and their waste of time and tax dollars.

Finally, once I left the NCI to work at Walter Reed Army Medical Center, and away from my "political" bosses…my paper was published in the *Journal of the National Cancer Institute* itself.

Fortunately, the journal is reviewed by non-government scientists independent of the NCI itself. And I was awarded the Young Research Investigator prize for this work at Walter Reed.

It wasn't until 2002 that there was finally general recognition among physicians that using RDA guidelines to treat diseases was not adequate. Thanks to the publication of a pair of papers by Fairfield and Fletcher in the *Journal of the American Medical Association*.[15]

The stage was finally set for accepting that nutrients should be taken in adequate doses and in natural combinations in order to prevent and cure diseases such as cancer. Three-quarters of a century after the British initiated their first efforts in the war on cancer.

Vitamin C breakthrough for cancer targets tumors at the source

Despite the best efforts of the Medical Mandarins at the National Institutes of Health, research on vitamin C and cancer HAS continued...And the results of several new studies have allowed me to bring a lot of thinking and observations from the past 35 years together. Into a rare—but very real—honest-to-goodness cancer breakthrough.

There has been a lot of interest in the ability of vitamins and minerals to lower the risk of cancer for many decades. But the way a lot of the research is done just doesn't get it right. They use the wrong nutrients, the wrong forms of administration, the wrong doses, for the wrong reasons. Then, if they don't find a positive result, the "experts" have been all too quick to say, "See, it doesn't work!"

Vitamin C has endured more than its share of this shoddy research and scientific bias. Especially when it comes to this nutrient's anti-cancer potential.

And thanks in large part to this inept research, many "experts" have been warning cancer patients against vitamin C for years.

When we began offering high-dose, intravenous vitamin C to cancer patients at Thomas Jefferson University Hospital 10 years ago, we first had to prove to a number of hospital review committees that it would be safe. (It was.) And that it wouldn't interfere with other treatments (chemotherapy and radiation). (It didn't.)

And now, a new toxicology study has been performed on intravenous vitamin C. And the results are very revealing.

The dose administered was 1 gram (1,000 mg) <u>per minute</u> over 4 consecutive days each week for a total of 4 weeks.[16]

That dose—1,000 mg—is more than the government's recommended <u>daily</u> allowance of vitamin C. And the subjects in this study got 1,000 mg every *minute*.

Researchers then determined how quickly vitamin C is eliminated from the body. They did this by finding the nutrient's "half-life." (Half-life means the time it takes for the concentration in the blood to be reduced by half. The radiation oncologists who burn out cancers are familiar with radioactive half-life.)

The half-life of vitamin C was measured as 2.0 hours (plus or minus, 36 minutes). In this sense you would think of vitamin C as "short-acting" if it were a drug. But the clearance time for all vitamin C to be eliminated from the body was 21 days, plus or minus 5 days.

I think a possible reason for this difference is that the body (particularly the muscles) acts as a reservoir for vitamin C—and can take up and store a large amount .

But it's important to note that <u>none of the study participants suffered any ill effects from this high-dose intravenous administration of vitamin C.</u>

This basic toxicology information is very important. (I wish my colleagues and I had been authorized to study vitamin C like this back in the 1980s instead of just looking at carotenoids. Although at least we were able to discover the importance of lutein and lycopene at the same time I was exposing the lack of any real evidence for beta-carotene. But I digress…)

The new study also tells us that it is probably impossible to achieve blood levels of vitamin C high enough to <u>treat</u> cancer by taking oral supplements.

IV vitamin C enhances chemo

So that answers the safety question about vitamin C for cancer patients. But what about the concerns regarding vitamin C's impact on other cancer treatments?

Well, new lab studies show that IV vitamin C actually *enhances* chemotherapy drugs like gemcitabine and erlotinib against pancreatic cancer cells (notoriously difficult to treat).[17] Researchers observed this effect even in cancer cells that are otherwise resistant to gemcitabine treatment.

This means doctors may be able to lower the doses of toxic chemotherapy drugs they give their patients if they also administer them with safe IV vitamin C.

So this new (and long overdue) research finally allows us to set aside old myths and misconceptions about administering vitamin C to cancer patients.

Of course, even after all of this has been settled, there will undoubtedly be the hardened skeptics who will refuse to believe it until someone answers the age-old question "but <u>how</u> does it work?"

Well, new scientific research now has that aspect covered too...

Not just an anti-oxidant

Early theories about the role of vitamin C (ascorbic acid) in preventing cancer focused on its role as an "anti-oxidant."

But oxidation and anti-oxidants are more complicated than it seems. It all goes back to Chemistry 101: Chemically, any oxidant can become an anti-oxidant, and any anti-oxidant can become an oxidizing agent, depending upon the surrounding molecular environment, acid-base balance, and other factors.

And this probably explains why test tube laboratory studies showed that high enough levels of vitamin C actually cause direct cancer cell death. When ascorbic acid gets so high, it may reverse action and become an oxidant, or may simply just act as an acid. Which poisons cells.

However, in lab studies, vitamin C was also effective against experimental tumors even at lower doses that could not kill cancer cells directly.

So, how does it work? Well, it turns out you don't have to kill cancer cells outright (and risk poisoning yourself).

Starve cancer cells to death

There is a two-stage model of cancer. (This model was key to my own PhD dissertation research, which recognized the importance of early childhood nutrition in the long-term risk of cancer.) The first stage involves some chemical damage that alters the DNA in normal cells, "mutating" them into individual cancer cells. This is called cancer initiation.

Then the cells have to grow into actual tumors. This stage is called cancer promotion. The ability of cancer tumors to grow (promotion) is based upon them hijacking the body's blood supply—which you know now as angiogenesis

And it now appears anti-angiogenesis is an important mechanism by which an agent can prevent cancer without having to actually kill the cells (which is the toxic property of today's cancer drugs). If you can prevent the cancer from getting blood supply, the cells will starve to death, without having to actually poison them.

And a convincing new study shows the anti-angiogenic properties of vitamin C. In fact, three of them.

A triple play against tumor growth

In lab models, researchers used an intravenous vitamin C dose of 25 to 60 grams.[18] (A dose you could safely get in 25 minutes to one hour with the "1-gram-per-minute" approach used in the human toxicity study reported above.)

First, the vitamin C inhibited endothelial (blood vessel) cells from multiplying—without harming normal, healthy endothelial cells. (Remember, chemotherapy drugs prevent cells from multiplying by poisoning normal cellular metabolism.).

Second, the vitamin C also decreased the migration of endothelial cells. This prevented new blood vessel cells from going to the cancer.

And, finally, the vitamin C prevented the endothelial cells from organizing into new blood vessel structures.

That's a triple play against cancer tumor growth.

Oral vitamin C supplements aren't enough to treat cancer

So, vitamin C turns out to be an "anti-angiogenic" powerhouse at doses that are very high, yet well-tolerated by humans. But it has to be administered intravenously to reach the doses that are safe and effective against cancer growth.

Now it's true there is a lot of evidence that lower oral doses of vitamin C (but still higher than the RDA) will *prevent* development of cancer in the first place. But you have to give vitamin C intravenously—directly into the bloodstream—to get high enough levels, long enough, to stop cancer once it is growing in the body. (So any "negative" studies using only oral doses to try to treat cancer don't really mean anything.)

This may sound extreme. But all cancer patients receive various intravenous therapies anyway. In fact, chemotherapy drugs are so toxic they have to be administered intravenously. If you swallowed them, they would poison and destroy the gastro-intestinal tract. Of course IV chemotherapy drugs cause enough physical devastation as it is (nausea, hair loss, fatigue, weakened immunity, another cancer—the list goes on). Intravenous vitamin C can be just as effective against cancer—if not more so. And it doesn't cause ANY of these toxic effects.

So you only have to ask yourself one question: which would you rather get?

Getting an IV vitamin C infusion is similar to having kidney dialysis—but much less invasive. You have to sit for awhile in the doctor's office while the nurse is monitoring and administering the infusion. At Thomas Jefferson University Hospital I set things up so that patients could also listen to mindfulness meditation oral exercises, visualization, and other mind-body approaches to make the time pass more pleasantly and productively.

The Clinical Laboratory Inspection Act governs the laboratories which formulate vitamin C intravenous infusions to ensure they are accurate, potent, and fresh. So look for a licensed physician that offers intravenous vitamin C infusion with an on-site certified laboratory.

Chapter 3

Natural treatments beyond vitamin C: An anti-angiogenesis arsenal

Vitamin E (alpha tocopherol)

It's important to note that natural vitamin E consists of four tocopherols and four tocotrienols. The reason for the mixed media on vitamin E is that the current cancer establishment insists on testing d-alpha tocopherol or dl-alpha tocopherol, both of which will not yield anti-cancer effects.

However, alpha tocopherol can neutralize the effects of certain cancer-causing compounds (such as N-nitrosamines). It may also stimulate the release of antitumor factors from the immune system. Animal studies suggest it can prevent some chemically induced cancers and it may reduce the size of tumors. One study, in humans, suggested a beneficial effect associated with the use of vitamin E in patients with superficial premalignant lesions in the mouth.

And it can be used in conjunction with some of today's more popular cancer treatments. It has been reported that a supplement of 800 mg per day of alpha-tocopherol, taken during radiation therapy for breast cancer, reduced side effects and improved general well-being.[19]

One of the best ways to work vitamin E into your diet is by enjoying a favorite fruit of mine. It's known around the everglades as "the alligator pear." You'll know it as the avocado. This fruit is jam-packed with vitamin E as well as 20 essential nutrients like fiber, potassium, B-vitamins, and folic acid.[20] And healthy essential fatty acids.

If you're going to supplement, I would recommend 100 IU of vitamin E per day.

The "Sun-Maid" Secret—Resveratrol

You may recognize the name of this plant compound for the "anti-aging" claims that are made. That may all be well and good, but there's a much more intriguing potential to resveratrol you may not hear elsewhere—it's potential to act against angiogenesis. This phytochemical compound is found in grape skins and grape seeds—and so in wine. In laboratory studies, it has shown anti-cancer effects by inhibiting the growth of over 12 different types of cancer cells, including prostate, breast, colon, pancreas, and ovarian carcinomas.[21]

Recently, resveratrol has been reported to be an angiogenesis inhibitor that is sufficiently potent in suppressing FGF-2 and VEGF-induced neovascularization *in vivo*.[22] Resveratrol has been shown to directly inhibit bovine endothelial cell proliferation, migration, and tube formation *in vitro*.[23]

In fact, resveratrol has the unique, balanced ability to provide either pro- or anti-angiogenesis effects depending upon the circumstances. In cancer, resveratrol has been shown to inhibit angiogenesis in tumors.[24]

The skin cancer savior—Genistein

This is a naturally occurring isoflavonoid found in soy products and certain other legumes like fava beans. It has been found to have anticancer activity in multiple tumor-cell types. In one study, genistein was found to inhibit angiogenesis in melanoma cells both in vivo and in vitro.[25] It has also been found to play a potential role in cervical cancer and prostate cancer. Epidemiological studies have shown there is an inverse relationship between dietary intake of genistein and cancer incidents, including breast, colon, and prostate cancer.[26]

A generally recommended dose is 50 mg per day. I recommend a brand called Bonistein ™ Genistein.

Curcumin

This powerful spice from India has been associated with dozens of health benefits by this point, as is usually the case with these natural wonders, but its anti-angiogenic properties are all but unsung.

More commonly known as turmeric, this spice has been used in Ayurvedic medicine for centuries and can serve as an antioxidant, analgesic, anti-inflammatory and antiseptic. Curcumin affects a variety of growth factor receptors and cell adhesion molecules involved in tumor growth, angiogenesis, and metastasis. In fact, curcumin is currently being examined specifically for effects on head and neck cancers, the sixth most common cancer worldwide.[27]

While the research still hasn't pinpointed an ideal dosage for fighting cancer, studies have used anywhere from 3,000 to 10,000 mg per day. A safe average dosage is 3,000 to 4,000 mg per day of a standardized supplement. Or, some recommend eating 1 teaspoon of turmeric per meal, more like a food quantity as a spice.

Fisetin

This naturally occurring pigment is found in many fruits, including strawberries, grapes, mangoes, and others as well as green tea. Recently, Indian researchers set out to determine if fisetin inhibits angiogenesis. The researchers first exposed endothelial cells to fisetin and found that it strongly inhibited the grown of endothelial cells and the ability of these cells to organize into new capillaries.

Even better, fisetin strongly suppressed production of two key regulators of angiogenesis: vascular endothelial growth factor and endothelial nitric oxide synthase.

All of this combined shows that fisetin inhibits angiogenesis both in vitro and in vivo and helps to squash many of the pro-angiogenic factors produced by cancer.[28]

Piperine

Piperine (*Piper nigrum*) is the compound in black pepper that gives it its kick. It has a long history of use in Ayurvedic and Southeast Asian medicine—used as a general restorative tonic. Piperine has been shown to substantially increase the body's ability to absorb the nutrients in foods and supplements. It has been shown to work a few different ways: by interfering with the body's ability to metabolize (or use up) substances, stimulating absorption of nutrients through the intestinal lining, and actually slowing down the action of the intestines in order to give the body more time to absorb the nutrients there. Similar to super-antioxidants that support other antioxidants, piperine can increase the effectiveness of other beneficial nutrients, including antioxidants enzymes.

Research has shown it can boost the bioavailability of cancer-fighter curcumin substantially. This is important, since curcumin is not easily absorbed by the body. In addition to these complementary effects, piperine has been shown to have direct antioxidant, anti-tumor, and anti-inflammatory properties.[29] A recent in vitro study showed piperine is able to directly stimulate immune cells.[30] And in recent tests on mice, piperine was shown to inhibit the spread of breast cancer cells in vitro and in vivo.[31]

A generally recommended dose is 20 mg per day of a brand called Bioperine® Piperine, which is a 50:1 standardized extract of Piper *nigrum* fruit.

And the list goes on...

These are just a few of the anti-angiogenic compounds we know about today. It's quite remarkable just how many researchers are finding—and with the growing list, it's becoming quite easy to integrate these compounds into your daily diet. Below is a list of some of the most readily accessible natural, anti-angiogenic compounds from foods and spices.

If you're concerned about cancer, one of the most important steps you can take is to load your plate, meal after meal, with a large variety of these anti-angiogenic foods. And be sure to experiment with the use of fresh herbs, to add even more protective benefits to each meal. And of course, keep them organic and pesticide-free if you can.

Fruits:
Apples, blackberries, blueberries, cherries, clementine tangerines, cranberries, grapefruit, lemons, nectarines, oranges, peaches, pomegranates, raspberries, red grapes, strawberries, and tomatoes.

Herbs & Spices:
Basil, black pepper, cilantro, cinnamon, cloves, cocoa powder, flaxseed, garlic, ginger, ginseng, lavender, licorice root, nutmeg, oregano, parsley, rosemary, tarragon, thistle, thyme, and turmeric.

Vegetables:

Artichokes, beets, bok choy (Chinese cabbage), broccoli, Brussels sprouts, red cabbage, carrots, cauliflower, chard, collard greens, endives, fennel, garlic, kale, mustard greens, olives, onions, peas, parsnips, peppers, pumpkins, radishes, salsify, scallions, shallots, soybean sprouts, spinach, string beans, sweet potatoes, tomatoes, turnips, watercress, and winter squash.

Mushrooms:

Enoki mushrooms, king oyster, maitake, matsutake, oyster mushrooms, reishi mushrooms, and shiitake.

Seafood:

Cuttlefish, flounder, haddock, halibut, herring, mackerel, oysters, salmon, sardines, sea cucumbers, seaweed, shrimp, sole, squid, squid ink, and tuna.

Legumes:

Almonds, cashews, chestnut, edamame, fava beans, lentils, lima beans, pine nuts, tofu, natto, and walnuts.

Beverages:

Apple cider, cocoa powder, coffee, green tea, miso, red wine, soy milk, and white wine.

You'll recognize many of these foods from the list of cancer preventive foods compiled by the British Empire Cancer Campaign of the 1920's and promoted as part of the Nazi War on Cancer during the 1930's. Decades later, the U.S. National Cancer Institute seized on their misunderstanding about beta-carotene as the "magic bullet" ingredient that explained the anti-cancer activity of these foods. But they missed the boat when it comes to the vitamins that are really important, and now we have the new evidence about the role of anti-angiogenesis factors in these foods.

The Tane Secret that could finally put Cancer in the Crosshairs

The story of what I call the *Tane Secret* (pronounced Tah-Neigh) is one of the most fascinating in all of natural medicine—and highlights a very important point about the true nature of scientific research.

As I've always said, for the truest advancements in medicine, *follow the science no matter where it leads.*

But what many researchers, doctors and certainly pharmaceutical shills often fail to see is that science will usually point to the past for some of the breakthroughs that will change our future.

A better name for a new revelation

So why *Tane*? Tane is the Polynesian god of nature and in an even broader sense, the god of good.

I feel it's a fitting name because as you'll see...this natural wonder that has been helping the peoples of the South Pacific for centuries, and is now astonishing scientists in the world's most modern laboratories. And yet, it *still* had its traditional name dragged through the mud for nearly a decade.

I'd like to do my small part in righting a huge medical wrong.

The Tane Secret revealed: Kava

Kava root extract is the medical secret that could revolutionize modern medicine. Its specific origin within the South Pacific is highly debated, but most recent work places the origin and domestication of kava (*piper methysticum*) on a tiny cluster of islands known as Vanuatu.[32]

Widely recognized as one of the premier unspoiled scuba diving destinations on the planet, and known traditionally for the daring "tower jumpers" who leap from great heights held back only by tree vines that let them fall within inches of the ground far below, Vanuatu may someday be better known as the birthplace of a true cancer prevention breakthrough.

Religion within the Polynesian culture is intertwined with many aspects of everyday life. Of course, when one thinks of far away South Pacific islands, the mind immediately recalls the famous heads first discovered on Easter Island by the Dutch in 1722.

These statues likely represent supreme chiefs, vital to the history and growth of this ancient civilization. Over 800 of them still stand on likely burial grounds and help exemplify the passed-down dedication to religion throughout the South Pacific.

Today, as a result of thousands of missionaries from Europe at the end of the 19th century, Christianity is the prevailing religion. However, whether it is the polytheism of sun gods and ocean gods or the monotheism of Christianity, kava has always persisted within the culture of the South Pacific.

What looks like an ordinary shrub, this hardy plant is fast-growing with multiple light to dark green stems. But the root system is its most-sought asset.

These roots (fresh or dried) are pulverized and brewed into a tea, traditionally used as a stress reliever, with many drinking it at the end of nearly every day. Forget about those fake "Polynesian" cocktails with the paper umbrellas—this is the real "Polynesian Cocktail Hour."

On the other side of the Pacific, the citizens of Vanuatu take their cultivation of kava very seriously. In fact, exportation is strictly regulated only to strains deemed as "noble" varieties. Their laws also mandate that exported kava must be cultivated at least five years and farmed organically.

I am up-to-date with the latest observations on traditional use of kava from my research associate who just came back from doing field work in the South Pacific.

New research in the 1980's changed everything

In 1985, *The Hawaii Medical Journal* baffled scientists by publishing a paper, the likes of which few scientists had ever seen before.

Just a few years prior, The South Pacific Commission Cancer Registry was formed. Its mission was to survey and monitor cancer rates for men and women throughout the Pacific Island nations. The researchers used Los Angeles Caucasians as a point of reference.

What it found absolutely confounded the commission.

Following are the cancer incidence rates per 100,000 males in the areas surveyed...

Los Angeles—307.2
Western Samoa—90.2
Fiji—75.0
Vanuatu—70.9[33]

For nearly a decade following the initial survey, medical professionals tried to figure out what could possibly be making such an impact on the citizens of these island nations. Their diets were analyzed, smoking rates were analyzed,[34] even the kind of tobacco commonly used was analyzed . And yet...researchers could not explain these incredibly low cancer rates.

Having done my own scientific field work in the South Pacific during the late 1970s, I had worked with many of these same researchers on other studies regarding diet and health in the Pacific during the 1980's and early 1990's.

The kava connection unfolds

As it turned out, just as the South Pacific Commission was completing their survey, statistics were being gathered for a growing industry within the South Pacific--the kava industry.

And when these two surveys were looked at side-by-side— cancer rates and kava consumption--a breakthrough correlation began to form.

In every country where both these figures were studied, the more kava consumed, the lower the cancer incidence.[35,36]

This inverse relation was measured in kilograms of kava consumed per year versus cancer incidence per 100,000 males.

So let's recap—the lung cancer rates in Fiji during the 1980's were 76 percent lower than those in Los Angeles at the time. In Vanuatu it was even lower -Seventy seven percent less.

And it appears one of the primary reasons may very well be this time-tested, culturally-renowned herbal tea.

So what happened? Why hasn't so much more already been accomplished on researching this time-tested, natural cancer breakthrough?

A tempest in a teapot...

Supplement sales for all kinds of herbs and vitamins began to really boom in the 1980's, and kava was no exception.

But before too long the brakes were slammed on operations amid a controversy which some still hotly debate to this day...

And new emerging science continuously calls the origin of this controversy into question.

Liver toxicity reports caused the United Kingdom's FDA counterpart to ban kava sales in the 1990's. Suddenly, the kava industry shrank by 50% and all of the promise behind kava and its active compound, *kavalactones* seemed to vanish from the mainstream.[37]

Luckily, botanical researchers kept its potential alive with bold new studies. The kava industry fought hard to clear its name, refuting the earlier studies that were using unproven and unverified forms of kava. And citing centuries of traditional use with no adverse reports.

In 2003, I asked leading European researchers to prepare a review of scientific studies showing the lack of toxicity of kava and published it in the premier volume of my scientific review journal, *Reviews in Integrative Medicine*, published by the same medical publisher as my leading textbook. That review found that observations on kava were confounded by patients taking prescription drugs that are toxic to the liver. It wasn't the herb that was at fault, it was the drugs!

But perhaps the strongest case for kava comes from the current crop of studies using verified kava, which show no adverse effects regarding liver toxicity.

And these studies are finally revealing kava's true potential…

20 years later—science finally prevails

The floodgates are now open and kava is finally prepared to take its place in the medical limelight. We could begin almost anywhere with this torrent of medical research. To date, over seven forms of cancer have been tested in preliminary studies, all with positive results.

Bladder cancer: Studies using mouse models performed at UC Irvine in 2002 and funded in part by the National Cancer Institute revealed an active component within kava, flavokawain A. Researchers found that flavokawain A encourages cell death in pre-cancerous cells by overcoming the effects of mutated proteins. This property is similar to a chemopreventative effect. All three bladder cancer mouse models responded well…and unsurprisingly, there was no evidence of toxicity from the falvokawain A.[38]

Bone cancer: Likewise, a report published in 2013 highlights another active component of kava, flavokawain B. This compound was shown to halt osteosarcoma cell lines and promote cell death. This was shown to be a chemotherapeutic and chemopreventive compound. In other words, it may help prevent *and* treat cancer.[39]

Colon cancer: An animal model designed to determine whether kava consumption reduces markers of colon cancer opened eyes even further in 2012. This 14-week trial revealed that kava-consuming groups had significantly fewer precancerous lesions compared to the control group. The results support that kava may help reduce colon cancer risk and that kava is safe to consume.[40]

Lung cancer: Another mouse-model study was conducted at the University of Minnesota. Researchers used a mouse model that is routinely used to predict lung cancer behavior in humans. The results were astounding. Researchers identified naturally occurring components of kava that appear to prevent the formation of up to 99% of cancer cell lines.[41]

One of the leading researchers called this research **"truly unprecedented in its potential impact."**

And all of this research is just the beginning…

What YOU can do now

It is great news that while medical research on kava went into a near 20-year hibernation period, the production of kava never did.

Traditionally, people in Fiji drink quite a bit of kava tea every day. It can add up to anywhere from 1 to 4 kg of kava per year. That comes out to a whopping 11,000 mg per day—essentially a small bucket-full of kava tea.

So a more practical approach, if you aren't able to incorporate so much of any tea into your daily life…would be to take a kava supplement along with drinking the tea. You can buy raw kava root and make your own tea at home. It's simple to do, but most American palettes might not find the flavor to their liking. For recipes, visit, www.gokava.com and visit their recipe page for teas, smoothies and even a French press recipe.

For use as an everyday supplement, I recommend at least 400 mg a day and always an organic, preferably grown in the South Pacific. To find a form that meets all of these requirements, visit www.herbal-island.com and look for their Kava Kava root extract.

Chapter 4

Antioxidants for prevention
of cancer cell formation

Vitamin C is probably the most well-known antioxidant, along with vitamins A, D, and E, and selenium. All of these are readily available and the research is extensive. However, the following are a few antioxidants you may not have heard of for fighting cancer.

The accumulation of free-radical ions at the cellular level is thought to trigger the process of carcinogenesis—the development of cancer cells. These free radicals are in the atmosphere and are formed by the ionizing effects of the sun. They can also come from external toxins, such as pesticides and other chemicals in our food. But they're also formed naturally as a byproduct of certain processes in the body.

Substances called antioxidants help keep free radicals in check, thus helping to prevent the formation of cancer cells. The body produces some antioxidants on its own. But you also get them from the foods you eat. Plants in the natural environment include a wide variety of potent antioxidants. Plants, like people, must protect themselves from the oxidative effect of free radicals in the atmosphere and from solar and other radiation.

Many plant compounds have been developed and tested for the ability to serve as antioxidants. In addition, various basic nutrients, such as vitamins, minerals, and amino acids have been found to have antioxidant properties. And when combined, antioxidant ingredients have been shown to work together to multiply their effects as a whole.

These findings are especially helpful if you or someone you love has undergone, or is undergoing mainstream treatments. Chemotherapy and radiation cause severe free-radical formation (oxidative stress) on the body. And while some oncologists have been concerned that antioxidant supplements may interfere with this type of cancer treatment, this has not been proven to be the case. Antioxidant supplements can help the body recover from the effects of cancer treatment as well as helping to prevent the recurrence of cancer.

Acetyl-L-Carnitine (ALC) is an amino-acid with antioxidant properties. ALC helps turn the nutrients in our food into energy for our cells. It can help you overcome fatigue and improves the function of the brain and nervous system. This can be very helpful for those recovering from cancer. It's also helpful to those suffering the effects of mainstream cancer therapies, such as the notorious "chemo-brain."[42] ALC has also been studied for its potential to help enhance the effects of traditional chemotherapy.[43] A generally recommended dose would be 1,000 mg per day.

Alpha Lipoic Acid (ALA) is an essential fatty acid that is critical for the body. ALA supports energy production inside the cells and is a powerful antioxidant. But it also has the unique ability to extend the life of other antioxidants like vitamins C and E— making it an antioxidant of antioxidants. This powerful antioxidant also happens to be both water- and fat-soluble. This means it can reach all parts of the body to help fight free radicals. Alpha-lipoic acid has been shown to have anticancer effects by activating glutathione peroxidase (another potent antioxidant in the body) and decreasing oxidative stress in cancer patients. One recent study found that ALA could initiate cell death in lung cancer cells.[44]

ALA is found primarily in animal sources, including red meat, liver, heart, and kidney. The most abundant plant sources include spinach, broccoli, tomatoes, Brussels sprouts, potatoes, peas, and rice bran. It has also been suggested that food intake reduces the bioavailability of ALA. So when supplementing, it is recommended that ALA be taken 30 min before or 2 hours after eating.[45] A generally recommended dose would be 300 mg per day.

Coenzyme Q10 is found in every cell in the body and is a powerful antioxidant. It plays a critical role in the process of turning food into energy for the cells. In the laboratory, coenzyme Q10 has been shown to prevent cancer and reduce cancer cell growth. It can also improve white blood cell and immune system function. One recent study has shown that coenzyme Q10 may provide much-needed protection to the heart when undergoing chemotherapy.[46] In a recent pilot study, researchers found that supplementing with coenzyme Q10 and additional antioxidant vitamins (vitamin C, selenium, folic acid, and others) could extend survival time in patients with end-stage cancer.[47] A generally recommended dose would be 150 mg per day.

Selenium is a powerful antioxidant, which means it helps protect against oxidative stress and free-radical damage. It is thought to work particularly well in partnership with vitamin E. Selenium also supports your immune system, helping to protect against infection. It also plays a part in human growth and development. Several studies show that the level of selenium in the food supply of a given population is related to their rate of cancer. The lower the selenium, the higher the risk of cancer.

In fact, I had the opportunity of serving as the principal co-investigator on a cancer prevention study using selenium in a county in China. This particular county (Qidong County, Jiangsu Province) had a particularly high incidence of liver cancer. We found that the areas that had low levels of selenium in the blood or in the locally available grains had a higher rate of liver cancer— and that by giving selenium supplements it is possible to raise selenium in blood to levels that prevent cancer.

Dietary selenium supplementation has also been shown to be effective in blocking the formation of chemically-induced tumors in the gastrointestinal tract, liver, breast, skin, and pancreas in laboratory animals. And in human clinical trials, dietary selenium supplementation has been shown to prevent skin cancer and lower the risk of other cancers.

Other studies have clearly shown protective effects of this trace element even when given after carcinogen exposure. Such results suggest that selenium owes at least part of its effects to a decrease in the spread of any cancer cells that form.

Remember to use caution when it comes to dosage

As I have warned before regarding recommended allowances, the cancer protection offered by selenium is generally observed at concentrations greater than those known to meet the requirements for normal growth and metabolic activity (i.e. the RDA). And, as observed with other nutrients, continuous intake of selenium is necessary for maximum inhibition of cancer.

However, while selenium toxicity is rare, it is a real concern. To avoid side effects and potential toxicity, it's best to keep selenium intake at or below 400 mcg per day. Organic forms of selenium, such as selenomethionine, are absorbed as well as sodium selenite salt, but can persist in the body longer and thus theoretically pose a higher risk of toxicity.

Chapter 5

Immune surveillance: detecting cancer before it strikes

Mainstream science bureaucrats continue to pour money into surgery, radiation, and chemotherapy. But the past still holds many promising answers. Better answers.

Fortunately, others outside the NCI science bureaucracy have embraced the possibilities. Many private institutions and independent scientists have provided a considerable amount of research on more positive approaches. These approaches are based on ancient knowledge and wisdom. But now, we are able to apply innovative, cutting-edge knowledge of how cells grow. This approach is actually way ahead of the curve when it comes to a new understanding of how the body works.

I have outlined a "triple-play" approach to fighting cancer. It focuses on three proven alternatives to the toxic triple approach of chemotherapy, radiation, and surgery. These proven approaches can help prevent and treat cancer, as well as improve the condition of cancer survivors. So far you've read about the power of anti-angiogenesis, and antioxidants. In this chapter, I will talk about the importance of immunity in fighting cancer.

In the 1960s, a leading group of researchers discovered a critical connection between the immune system and cancer. They found that strengthening the immune system can help prevent and fight cancer. This is now a cornerstone of a natural approach. (As opposed to standard cancer treatments that are actually harmful to the immune system and to other healthy human cells.)

Cancer cells are actually formed continuously throughout the body due to the presence of free-radical ions that damage our cells. A healthy immune system can actually recognize these abnormal cancer cells. Once an abnormal cell is spotted, the immune system sends out "Natural Killer" cells (NK cells). These NK cells eliminate the cancer cells before they can grow into actual tumors.

Pro-immune effects of natural products include both enhancing the immune system's immune surveillance system (like a "distant early warning" defense system) as well as stimulating the Natural Killer cells that eliminate cancer cells as they form in the body.

Following are some of the most important nutrients for supporting the immune system and fulfilling the need for immune surveillance in the fight against cancer. Of course, there are many, many more. But these are most readily available and have the research to support them as well. Many of these may also act in other ways, but their overall impact on immune health is substantial, and it's essential they not be overlooked.

Vitamin C (ascorbic acid) is one of the most effective antioxidants. However, research has shown it may have an overall profound effect on the immune system. This was apparent even in the early cancer research uncovered by my colleague at the NIH (as noted above). Where it was not only shown to help cut off the power source of the tumors, but actually stops the formation of unhealthy cells. But unfortunately, thanks to the complete misdirection of the NIH, the research on all the potential mechanisms of action of vitamin C is still lacking.

Epidemiological evidence shows that populations who eat diets high in vitamin C have a lowered risk for some cancers. This may be because of the antioxidant function of vitamin C and its ability to block the formation of N-nitrosamines (cancer-causing substances formed in the stomach from certain foods). A strong epidemiological finding has been the association between high intakes of foods rich in vitamin C and a reduced risk of stomach cancer. There is a weaker link to a decreased risk of cervical cancer in smokers. In other research, it may also help counteract the toxicity of some conventional cancer treatments while enhancing the cell-killing effect of others.[48]

A protective effect of ascorbic acid in colorectal cancer could exist by its prevention of fecal nitrosamines or against other fecal mutagens. In addition, a mechanism has been proposed whereby vitamin C inhibits DNA synthesis and spread of preneoplastic cells. Administration of ascorbic acid has been shown to produce a 30–40% increase in protective enzymes.

Studies of rectal polyps among patients with a family history, support the possibility of a protective effect of vitamin C in polyp formation and thus possibly in colorectal cancer. With 400 mg of vitamins C and E administered to patients following polypectomy, after 2 years, the recurrence data rate was reduced approximately 20%.[49]

Ascorbic acid is generally tolerated well, but at high doses it may cause stomach irritation, heart-burn, nausea, vomiting, drowsiness, and headaches. Some oncologists are concerned that high-dose vitamin C may alter the absorption and excretion of some drugs used in the treatment of cancer, and may interfere with radiation therapy. However, there are no clinical studies documenting such effects. In adults, there is significant anecdotal evidence that vitamin C is safe at dosages of 1,000 mg per day and very minimal toxicity has been reported even at much higher dosages. However, there are few controlled studies of the toxicity of vitamin C.

Major proponents of high-dose vitamin C for cancer treatment included the late Nobel laureate Dr. Linus Pauling and Dr. Ewan Cameron. And while their research would need to be confirmed by more rigorous studies, they did provide a number of observational reports, case studies, and pilot studies involving large numbers of advanced cancer patients. These patients were given high doses of vitamin C. They reported that it appeared to improve overall wellbeing and quality of life, as well as resulted in a significant increase in the survival of patients with various types of advanced cancer.[50] High-dose vitamin C levels can be achieved through intravenous infusion under direct medical supervision, as well as oral administration.

For my last act, while serving as Executive Director of the Center for Integrative Medicine at Thomas Jefferson University Hospital, I fought and won through all the hospital professional, pharmacy, and safety committees to gain approval to offer high dose vitamin C infusions right in this major university hospital under direct medical supervision for patients recovering from cancer and cancer therapy.

A generally recommended dose is 750 mg per day, in combination with other "triple-play" nutrients (see Chapter 6) as a dietary supplement; and high-dose IV under direct medical supervision.

Vitamins B1, B2, B3, B5, B6, B12. Most people have heard of B vitamins. But do you know what they can actually do for you? The B vitamins help optimize metabolism at the cellular level. Meaning, they are essential for energy of the cells. The B vitamins also play a role in many critical functions of the body. But they have also been shown to stimulate the immune system and inhibit cancer cell formation. Significant data suggest that a deficiency of vitamin B12 or folic acid may actually lead to increased tumor development. A study published in *Cancer Epidemiology Biomarkers & Prevention* in 1999 reported an association of low levels of B12 with breast cancer in postmenopausal women.[51] Another study published in the *Annals of Internal Medicine* in 1998 has shown a protective effect of dietary folate against the development of colon cancer.[52] A generally recommended dose of vitamins B1, B2, B3, B4, B5, and B6 is 100 mg of each per day. For B12, a generally recommended dose is 1 mg (or 1,000 mcg) per day in combination with other "triple-play" nutrients.

Zinc and calcium. Zinc, together with other minerals, like calcium, is thought to have a role in inhibiting cancer growth through enhancement of the immune system and/or by direct effects on the cells. Zinc, an essential constituent of numerous enzymes, functions in cell replication and tissue repair. Calcium plays an important role in many cell functions including the overall survival of the cell. It helps control cell proliferation and synthesis of DNA. Investigations found that supplementing with 1,250 mg of calcium per day significantly reduced cell proliferation in patients at high risk for large bowel cancer.[53] Epidemiological studies support the hypothesis that a higher calcium intake may reduce risk for colon cancer. One large study showed that people who took calcium supplements of 1,200 mg per day showed a decreased risk of colorectal polyps.[54] A generally recommended dose for zinc is 250 mg per day and for calcium it's 2,000 mg per day.

Lentinen and other mushroom extracts. Lentinen is a plant compound extracted from shiitake and other mushrooms. It has been shown to have potent anti-cancer properties, similar to other mushroom extracts. Mushrooms, such as shiitake, used for cancer in traditional Asian medicine, appear to contain a substance called polysaccharides. These polysaccharides appear to activate the immune system NK cells. In addition, some mushroom extracts have been shown in the laboratory to directly kill cancer cells, but leave normal cells alone. These observations have been made with mushrooms that are edible, such as shiitake, maitake, and gandoderma.

A study from Korea, including 272 patients, found that the higher the intake of mushrooms, the lower the prevalence of gastric cancer. In another study, 68 patients with advanced, non-small cell lung cancer were given a polysaccharide peptide mushroom isolate. This was a randomized, placebo-controlled, double-blind study. Patients in the intervention group showed stimulation of the immune system.[55]

Some polysaccharides from mushrooms may also help protect bone marrow from the harmful effects of chemotherapy and may have clinical application in recovering from cancer. Clinical trials are under way in Japan evaluating the use of mushrooms as adjunctive therapy to chemotherapy. The National Cancer Center Research Institute of Japan conducted a 15-year epidemiological study from 1972 to 1986. They looked at the cancer rates in close to 175,000 people. They found that mushroom farmers had overall lower cancer death rates when compared to non-farmer populations (160.1 per 100,000 compared to 97.1 per 100,000).[56]

A generally recommended dose of lentinen is 2,000 mcg (or 2 mg) from shiitake mushroom with a 4:1 extract of Lentinus edodes, caps and stems (equivalent to 8 mg of dried mushroom).

Vitamin D. A new research review looked at the results of 25 separate studies that measured vitamin D levels in 17,332 people at the time of their cancer diagnosis. Higher vitamin D levels were linked to significantly better survival rates for people with breast or colon cancer or lymphoma. There was also a positive effect for lung, stomach, prostate, and melanoma skin cancers, as well as leukemia.[57]

In addition, a recent study that showed that women with breast cancer who had higher vitamin D levels had double the survival rate of women with lower levels.

And this result was in a population where the "high" vitamin D group of women actually just had "sufficient" levels of the vitamin. Imagine if all women were at the truly optimal levels shown by research to be most beneficial to their health?

I recommend a dose of 5,000 IU per day of vitamin D.

Chapter 6
COMBINED EFFECTS:
Double- and triple-plays with these fabulous five additional ingredients

In addition to vitamin C, the following five additional ingredients have the unique power to address two or all three critical cancer-fighting effects. They provide **antioxidant protection, immune support, and have anti-angiogenesis** effects.

The yellow spice breakthrough:
Curcumin (Curcuma longa).

Curcumin is the gold-colored curry spice commonly used in India. It has been used for centuries as a spice in foods (turmeric) and as an herbal remedy in India, Malaya, and Southeast Asia. But it has suddenly been "discovered" by modern science leading to a torrent of current research. Curcumin has been extensively researched as a treatment for cancer. Its antioxidant effects are 10 times stronger than that of vitamin E. And it has been shown to stop tumor growth.

In a review of over 728 curcumin analogs which covers the literature from 1815 to mid-2009, researchers showed that curcumin interfered with multiple cell signal pathways including the spread of cancer cells, angiogenesis, and inflammation.[58] Therefore, among the national products shown to possess chemical preventive and anticancer properties, curcumin is one of the most potent.

Other recent research has shown that curcumin can help stop the spread of cancer (metastasis) by decreasing the invasiveness of cancer cells in a lung cancer model.[59] It has also been shown to have a direct effect against cancer cells in colon cancer, chronic lymphocytic leukemia, liver cancer and ovarian cancer. And can slow the spread of melanoma, prostate cancer, multiple myeloma, lymphoma, and others.

In one recent study, curcumin was found to be lethal to human bladder cancer cells. It induced cell death and stopped the spread. The effect of curcumin was shown to be stronger than that of cisplatin (a common chemotherapy drug).[60]

Curcumin has also been shown to have the unique ability to help enhance the effectiveness of chemotherapy when it may otherwise fail. Multidrug resistance to anticancer drugs is a major cause of chemotherapy failure for patients. Curcumin may be used as a chemo sensitizer to make tumor cells more sensitive to the effects of chemotherapy.[61] Thus potentially lowering the effective dose of toxic chemotherapy—an example of true complementary medicine.

Studies have shown it to exhibit similar activities to those drugs that have been developed to block tumor necrosis factor, vascular endothelial cell growth factor, human epidermal growth factor, and HER2.

A generally recommended dose is 200 mg per day as a dietary supplement, although dietary intake can be higher when used as a food spice versus a supplement.

The pungent protector: Garlic (Allium sativa).

Unlike many other herbs, garlic, is also a biologically active food with presumed medicinal properties, including possible anti-cancer effects. Garlic has been found to possess over 100 constituent compounds. Some have been looked at individually, but one can't discount the potential importance of the benefits of the whole.

Clinical studies of garlic in humans address several areas including protective associations with cancer as well as clinical adverse effects. There are multiple clinical studies with promising but some conflicting results. Some data, primarily from case-control studies, suggest dietary garlic consumption is associated with decreased risk of laryngeal, gastric, colorectal, and endometrial cancer, and colon polyps.

Recent research has found that the allicin in garlic (the main ingredient in garlic that gives it its distinctive flavor) can stimulate cell death via various actions.[62]

In a population-based, case-control study conducted in Shanghai, China, investigators found a link between the intake of allium vegetables, including garlic, scallions, onions, chives, and leeks, and the risk of prostate cancer. Men in the highest of three intake categories of total allium vegetables (more than 10.0 grams per day) had a statistically significantly lower risk of prostate cancer than those in the lowest category (less than 2.2 grams per day). Similar comparisons between categories showed reductions in risk for men in the highest intake categories for garlic and scallions.[63]

You can increase your garlic intake by adding it to your taste to any vegetable, fish, or meat dish. One to two cloves per day is recommended. If supplementing with a garlic extract, a generally recommended dose is 200-400 mg, two to three times per day.

The "back from the brink" cancer weapon: Sutherlandia frutescens ("Cancer Bush")

In my explorations of the silent cures of South Africa, Sutherlandia frutescens is regarded as one of the most potent. It has had a long but hidden history of use as a safe and effective remedy for various health conditions by all cultures in the region. It has long been used as a supportive treatment in cancer, hence one of its common names—"Cancer Bush." It is called *Kankerbos* in Afrikaans, a dialect of the Dutch settlers. And in the indigenous *Tswana* tongue, as in Botswana, it is called *"Phetola"* which means "it changes." And indeed the plant changes the course of many illnesses for the better.

Sutherlandia has traditionally been used for enhancing wellbeing, immune support, longevity, stress, depression and anxiety. It was one of the few treatments found useful during the deadly global "Spanish Flu" epidemic after WW I that killed 20 million people worldwide during 1918-19. It works by helping the body heal and restore a normal state of health (or homeostasis) by mobilizing its own resources to overcome many physical and mental stresses. Research studies show that is works broadly among the body systems. This indicates that it functions as an *adaptogen*, as well as an immune stimulant. Studies also indicate significant antioxidant activity, another important anti-cancer property.

Cancer bush contains a substance called *L-canavanine*. This potent compound has been shown to stop pancreatic cancer cells in their tracks.[64] Cancer bush also contains GABA, which has been shown to stamp a "cease and desist" on tumor cells.[65] And clinical trials are now underway testing it against the immune system's ultimate enemy, the AIDS virus.[66]

But beyond the technical aspects of this wonder-find, there lies a mysterious aspect that could make it the "back from the brink" cancer weapon patients have been praying for. And that's the ability of the cancer bush to halt the deadly "wasting" process that so many terminally ill patients experience. This wasting away is called *cachexia*.

The presence of cachexia in cancer patients has long been understood to mean that cancer is a metabolic disorder, systemically throughout the body, rather than being just the presence of a malignant tumor. Therefore, a natural product like Sutherlandia, which also acts as an adaptogen, can show potential benefits over an approach to just killing cancer cells. Accordingly, it functions as an appetite stimulant in wasted patients, but not in healthy people. Dr. Credo Mutwa, one of South Africa's most respected healers, has seen patients who weighed as little as 57 lbs turn the tides and reach 100 lbs. in just 7 months.[67]

A generally recommended dose is 600 mg per day of *Sutherlandia frutescens* leaf extract.

The Mother's Day cancer crusher: Chrysanthemum

Chinese medicine also offers complex mixtures of active herbal remedies for cancer. One interesting and important ingredient is

Chrysanthemum. Chrysanthemum is better known in the West as a simple decorative, hardy flowering plant. But the chrysanthemum itself is full of at least 15 different active and potent phytochemicals. Many of these phytochemicals act as pesticides to discourage predators, so it's not surprising that it would contain compounds that have anti-cancer properties. It is also a hardy plant, well known for its ability to withstand cold and continue to bloom even after other plants have closed down for the autumn and winter.

Chrysanthemum is a powerful symbol in Chinese and Japanese culture. It is often used as a tea in ceremonial occasions. Often a plant that is revered for its symbolic or iconic significance also has constituents that are very powerful herbal remedies. I recognized this common property of medicinal plants early in the development of medical anthropology in the early 1980's.[68]

Scientifically, Chrysanthemum morifloriam flowers have demonstrated various anti-cancer effects specifically against prostate cancer.[69] In Chinese medicine it is used for prostate cancer and prostate health together with reishi mushroom (*Ganoderma*), licorice root (*Glycyrrihiza glabra*), saw palmetto (*Serenoa repens*), and the adaptogen Sanchi Ginseng (*Panax pseudoginseng*).

Chrysanthemum and seven other active natural products were once available in the traditional Chinese combination remedy known as PC-SPES. In one of their rare, but still misguided, attempts to test a truly innovative approach to cancer, the NIH unwittingly used contaminated PC-SPES and had to halt their study, wasting more taxpayer dollars and a golden opportunity to expand the cancer treatment frontier. As a result of the contamination of the PC-SPES being tested, it was pulled off the market and is no longer available. Which is a shame, considering it was exceptionally effective. Particularly for re-differentiation, or returning cancerous cells back to a normal, healthy state.

However, similar, equally promising formulations made by different companies are now available. Chrysanthemum is included in a formulation called PC-CARE.

Treatment with PC-CARE or similar formulations should be individually monitored and sought from a qualified and knowledgeable traditional Chinese medical practitioner. Such practitioners may be found in Chinatowns in major urban areas and even some modern university hospital settings in the U.S.

The Middle-Eastern marvel: Black cumin (Nigella sativa)

Black cumin (*Nigella sativa*) is an annual flowering plant found in South and Southwest Asia. It is also called fennel flower, nutmeg flower, Roman coriander, black caraway seed, or black coriander, and sometimes onion seed or black seed. It is regarded as one of the greatest of all medicinal herbs in Islam. Modern research is actively investigating its anti-cancer properties. An extract has recently been found to be effective against pancreatic cancer in the laboratory. Pancreatic cancer is a notoriously difficult cancer to treat. So the potential of black cumin is giving researchers hope in finally finding an effective natural remedy.

Researchers at the Kimmel Cancer Cancer at Thomas Jefferson University in Philadelphia, with whom I used to work, have found that thymoquinone, an extract of nigella sativa seed oil, blocked pancreatic cancer cell growth and killed the cells by enhancing the process of programmed cell death. Using a human pancreatic cancer cell line, researchers found that adding thymoquinone killed approximately 80 percent of the cancer cells, but presumably without the toxic side effects of chemotherapy.[70]

Black cumin seed supplements are available in some natural food stores, vitamin shops, and from online supplement retailers. A good general dose is 500 mg per day.

Chapter 7

The business of cancer: How more cancer screenings and the uptick in diagnoses are doing more harm than good

Few things in life are more frightening than a cancer diagnosis. Just hearing the words, "You have cancer," can throw a person into a devastating tailspin—taking their loved ones along with them.

So imagine hearing those words when they're not actually true. Imagine having your life turned upside-down and facing mortality eye-to-eye, only to find out what you have isn't really cancer… it's a case of *mistaken identity*, or *false labeling*.

That's just what's happening to countless people around the country every day. They are receiving the shocking and demoralizing news that they have cancer—a life-threatening illness—when they actually have something that has no chance of ever killing them.

Not all "cancer" is created equal

So how is this happening? It all comes down to what you call things, and our medical establishment has taken to calling things "cancer" even when they're not.

In dermatology, for instance, pathologists have long observed relatively benign tumors as only "Grade ½" based on the benign appearance of the cells. Normally cancer cells are graded on a scale of one to four, so a half-grade is meant to register that cells don't really look like cancer—and they don't behave like it either.

But instead of just removing these skin growths and letting their patients go on with their day, dermatologists put the fear of death in them by calling them cancer. (As it is, they already get a lot of practice putting the fear of death into their patients when it comes to the sun). The truth is most skin cancers are relatively benign growths and do not cause long-term problems if they're removed.

So why call these growths that don't even meet the pathological requirements for the lowest level—Grade 1—cancer?

Even the National Cancer Institute (NCI) is starting to wake up to this problem. A working group they recently sanctioned just advised the medical community that the "use of the term *cancer* should be reserved for describing lesions with a reasonable likelihood of lethal progression if left untreated."

Translation? If it can't kill a person, STOP calling it cancer!

The far-reaching effects of cancer scares

These unnecessary cancer diagnoses have effects far beyond the initial scare. Many cancers are being treated that don't need to be. And as we all know, treatment isn't benign in itself.

For those "Grade ½" skin lesions, treatment is simple (removal with local anesthetic, if that). But for other so-called "cancers," people are put through major surgery, toxic chemotherapy, and/ or radiation.

Take prostate cancer, the most common cancer in men. As men get older, they become more likely to develop an "occult cancer" of the prostate. But in most cases, this "cancer" is so slow-growing and silent that it never causes problems. In fact, if it's not discovered by overeager screening, it probably will go unnoticed—unless it shows up as an "incidental" finding at an autopsy of a man who has died in advanced old age of some other cause. If such a cancer is caught, however, you can count on aggressive, invasive and unnecessary treatment, not to mention mental anguish.

Cancer treatments remain among the most toxic, dangerous treatments still practiced anywhere since the Middle Ages—with many side effects of their own. They can even cause secondary cancers. *So the cancer you went in for won't kill you, but here's another one that probably will!*

When I was a medical resident, my next-door neighbor in Philadelphia was a retired fireman who came down with lymphoma.

He was treated with a new "miracle" cancer drug, Adriamycin (a chemotherapeutic agent originally developed from algae in the Adriatic Sea). He was cured of the cancer, but the Adriamycin destroyed his heart muscle and he quickly died—albeit "cancer-free." Knowing what we now know, I suspect the drug totally destroyed the cellular respiration function in the mitochondria, causing the heart to go first.

That's just one story, but there are lots more like it. And beyond its effects on individuals like my neighbor, this "over-diagnosis/ over-treatment crisis" makes us less healthy as a society.

Just think of the epidemic of vitamin D deficiency that has resulted from our being kept out of the sun for fear of skin cancers (91 percent of which don't really behave like cancer at all).

We now realize that lack of vitamin D can contribute to other, typically more serious, cancers (and heart disease, and respiratory diseases, and more).[71] So again, we're trading a relatively minor health concern for a major one.

Of course, the over-diagnosis/ over-treatment crisis wouldn't be possible without another, equally problematic aspect of modern oncology.

Cancer screening paves the way for problems

The concept of cancer screening in the United States has become highly problematic over the past three decades. For example, the medical establishment pushes dangerous, expensive and overused procedures such as colonoscopy (see Chapter 9), while virtually ignoring screening for lung cancer which causes far more cancer deaths.

Then, added to that, screening is identifying more of what doctors have been calling "early cancers," but which we now realize are not cancers at all. From a distance, it looks like the system has been catching more cancers and preventing more deaths due to cancer. But these statistics are misleading if the additional cancers were not going to cause death in the first place. It's all part of the statistical trickery used to create the illusion of some progress in the "war on cancer."

This numbers game makes us think we're getting ahead of cancer. But all we are really doing is just diagnosing more "non-cancers" and calling it a success when they don't kill us.

Here's an example: Breast cancer screening has led to an overall increase in incidence of new "cases," because both cancers and non-cancers are being detected. So when cancer death rates stay the same or decrease, despite a supposed increase in incidence, it allows the government to claim a false sense of victory.

The same is happening with prostate cancer and others.

And all the while, the real goal—to reduce the rates of late-stage cancers and cancer deaths—remains elusive.

Screening practices and programs designed for that purpose have not met their goals. All we have done is to increase detection of "early-stage" cancer but without any decline in "late-stage" cancer. If cancer is defined as a disease that will lead to death if untreated, then detecting an "early" cancer that would have never led to death is not detecting cancer at all.

And we have accomplished nothing.

When does screening make sense?

We need to understand and appreciate the biology of different cancers. If a cancer is very *fast-growing*, then no screening can realistically be effective when it comes to the population as a whole. If it is *slower-growing*, as with colon polyps that take a long time (15 years on average) to develop into colon cancer, then less frequent screening can be effective.

If growth is *very slow* (for example, exceeding human life expectancy, such as "occult" cancer of prostate) then screening is actually harmful because it detects lesions that need not and *should not* be treated.

The one unqualified success story we've seen with screening is for cervical cancer. Cervical cancer used to be one of the top causes of cancer deaths in women. But from 1955 to 1992, the cancer death rate has declined by almost 70 percent—thanks to widespread, easy, and effective screening.[72] No other cancer screening has shown anywhere near these kinds of positive results.

Given this sad state of affairs, what else is the NCI-approved panel I mentioned above proposing?

A common-sense solution

The practice of oncology in the United States is in serious need of a host of reforms to address the problems of over-diagnosis and over- treatment.

The advisory panel laid out a plan for dealing with this problem. First, as I mentioned earlier, it specifically advised that a number of "pre-malignant" conditions should no longer be called "cancer." This includes the common intra-ductal carcinoma of the breast (within the breast ducts) and even "high-grade" intraepithelial neoplasia of the prostate.

Instead, a different category of growth or tumor should be recognized and labeled appropriately as "non-cancer." Doesn't that sound less frightening? The panel suggests using such terms as "indolent lesions of epithelial origin" or IDLE.

A big part of the problem is all the medical sub-specialties involved in cancer. Each has its own terminology largely based upon the technologies they use, rather than a fundamental understanding of the biology of cancer. The use of new tools for diagnosing or treating diseases has driven the creation and practice of different medical specialties, each of which has developed exclusive uses of these technologies. This state of affairs calls to mind the admonition, "If your only tool is a hammer, then you see every problem as a nail."

Another result of medical sub-specialization is the different terminologies in use across the spectrum of pathology, radiology, surgery, and other medical specialties as well as the general community.

The panel has recommended that a body such as the Institute of Medicine determine what we should call these lesions now called cancer.

Then—in order to actually affect the rates of late-stage cancers and cancer deaths—all the other "pre-malignant" lesions must be tracked separately by government statisticians, instead of being lumped together with cancer. That's the only way we'll get an accurate view of what is and is not causing real cancer. This would vastly improve the quality of our cancer statistics, on which our national health policies are based.

Another proposal focuses on reducing over-diagnosis by reducing the use of low-yield diagnostic tests, reducing the frequency of screenings, focusing on high-risk populations, and raising requirements for taking a biopsy.

Finally, the panel recommended alternatives to treatment by focusing on the environment in which tumors arise. Strategies such as diet or chemoprevention (reducing the risk of cancer by specific micronutrient vitamins and minerals) may be as effective, and are less toxic, than traditional therapies.

Of course, given misplaced priorities for cancer research funding, the oncology community still has a long way to go before understanding the right doses, forms, and micronutrients to use. But some research is beginning to emerge that may point us in the right direction.

How the government could prevent 12,000 lung cancer deaths per year, but won't

One out of 10 smokers gets lung cancer. And those who smoke the most are most at risk.

But, two years ago, U.S. researchers found a simple way to prevent lung cancer among those highest at risk. And government science-bureaucrats refuse to acknowledge it.

Instead, we just hear the endless preaching about smoking cessation. But, in fact, most people who get lung cancer today are *former smokers*. They've already quit. But they're still getting lung cancer.

What do we tell <u>them</u>?

Plus, even as smoking goes down, people are still getting lung cancer. And the number of *non-smokers* with lung cancer is on the rise. In fact, one out of 100 non-smokers gets lung cancer, without ever taking a puff. But the government doesn't talk about these statistics. And you don't hear about this troubling fact in the news at all.

While driving through upstate New York last fall I heard a heartbreaking radio broadcast about a rally to raise public awareness for the 50,000 women with lung cancer in the U.S. who never smoked at all. They feel completely abandoned.

And what do we tell these women? They can't stop smoking because they never started. What causes their cancer? And how can they prevent it?

We stopped doing routine annual chest x-rays long ago because they really didn't detect new occurrences of cancer. And the risk of radiation was not worth it. Plus, x-rays have become old hat.

Instead, hospitals spend fortunes installing expensive, new imaging facilities. They even offer "open access" MRIs and CAT imaging equipment in freestanding, "walk-in" facilities–all to make more money.

Unfortunately, we give these expensive high-tech scans to folks with lower back pain–instead of to those at risk for lung cancer. The lower-back pain patients would be better off skipping the scan anyway. And going straight to physical therapy.

Meanwhile, the folks at risk for lung cancer are given nothing to believe in but the flimsy "smoke-and-mirrors" smoking cessation statistics.

And that's a crying shame, because preventative scans could clearly help reduce their risk…

Two years ago, the National Lung Cancer Screening Trial made this important discovery. The researchers found that screening high-risk smokers and ex-smokers with annual CAT scans would prevent 12,000 lung cancer deaths per year. These high-resolution x-rays can spot suspicious lung nodules.[73]

One of the study authors told Reuters, "This is the first paper that attempts to assess the impact of screening on lung cancer cases nationally."[74]

But why is this only the first paper on this huge health problem?

Why don't we screen for lung cancer?

My old colleague, Larry Kessler, studies the diagnostic value of screening and he recently published an editorial, which accompanied the new study in the journal *Cancer*. He said this new study is a "pivotal event that should have woken people up."

It should have, Larry. But it didn't.

The government and the medical profession prefer wagging politically correct fingers against smokers. And even against former smokers and non-smokers.

One-hundred-and-sixty thousand people die each year of lung cancer. That figure is higher than deaths caused by auto accidents, Vietnam, and most other cancers combined.

So, remind me again, why don't we screen for lung cancer?

But wait, the science bureaucrats in Bethesda have their reason why not.

The Division of Cancer Prevention at NCI–which hasn't gotten anything right in the last 30 years that I know about–says the numbers would not translate in the "real world" because those naughty smokers would not *want* to be screened!

Really–this is the *sole* reason why we don't screen them?

Can you hear those wagging fingers slicing through all the stifling hot air in Bethesda as you read this? Let's just keep punishing those naughty, politically incorrect smokers!

First of all, when are the political science creatures at NCI ever concerned with–or even aware of–the real world of average Americans? I doubt anyone gleefully schedules a colonoscopy or a Pap smear. But they do it because the NCI says they should.

The NCI also points to problems with screenings in general–such as costs and false positives–to discredit lung cancer screening. But those same problems apply to every single kind of screening. Mammograms. Pap Smears. Colonoscopies. They're all prone to the same problems. But the government still pushes them. Including many that are worthless, or worse.

What an incredibly, stupendously stupid comment from the agency that pushes cancer screening at every other opportunity! By the way, NCI gave up on finding cures for lung cancer long ago in favor of the anti-smoking mantra.

If you did not think that there is still gross, government-wide, politically correct discrimination against some people who get lung cancer–smokers and even the thousands of innocent, non-smokers–this should prove it to you.

Usually the government loves to find "victims" for everything. But the government has no love for victims of lung cancer. But remains happy to collect their cigarette taxes for this legal substance.

Unfortunately the government refuses to budge in their ignorance to real science. Because if they did, maybe they'd be clued in to the dangers of screenings they actually advocate for... like the ones you'll read about in the next chapters.

Ten medical procedures you may do better without!

Hundreds of thousands of Americans are injured, poisoned, and killed each year by modern medical technologies. Even the most respected medical journals and institutions have confirmed in various reports over the past 10 years the failures of American "modern medicine." Including deaths from unnecessary surgery, medication errors, clerical errors, hospital- acquired infections, and even from the "expected" negative side effects of drugs. All the while, health care costs are spiraling out of control and insurance companies are requiring patients to pay a greater share of the cost.

So despite all our breakthrough technology, American medicine often appears to be doing more harm than good. In fact, you may be surprised at what can be done without it!

It's time to rethink some of the medical myths and rituals that result in millions of useless tests, procedures, and "interventions" that appear to do more harm than good. Besides the huge waste of time and money they represent.

And now the American Board of Internal Medicine Foundation is doing just that with a new project called "Choosing Wisely." The foundation consists of doctors from nine of the top medical societies in the U.S. And the Choosing Wisely program has identified 45 different medical procedures that are of little or no value, from tests, to surgeries, and even commonly prescribed medications. Below I'll review the most commonly performed tests that are now considered inappropriate. Removing this kind of waste and abuse from the healthcare system could save billions of dollars a year.

Even the benefit of the routine yearly "checkup" is being questioned for most patients now. As reported in a New York Times article, back in 1979 a Canadian government task force recommended giving up the standard top-to-bottom annual physical exam.[75] They said it was "inefficient, nonspecific" and even "potentially harmful." That Canadian diagnosis was made the same year I graduated from a U.S. Ivy League medical school where we all sincerely believed the annual "checkup" was just practicing good medicine!

But the potential danger or harm of unneeded exams is that they may show "false positives," potentially lead to risky procedures and treatments, and/or more tests, which leads to more of the same. It's a vicious cycle. And every step along the way comes with the potential for harm. The controversy over the PSA test to try to detect prostate cancer is a good example.

But from the first day out of medical school, there remains a lot of simple inertia about what doctors expect they should be doing for their patients, and about what patients expect from their doctors. Not to mention all the economic incentives from the health care industry to provide more "care" whether needed or not.

There are also perverse incentives in medical research to discover more and more "biomarkers" for screening and "early detection" of diseases like cancer, despite the repeated abject failures of this approach for decades. And now, the new Director of the National Cancer Institute, Dr. Harold Varmus (a past director of the NIH) is back like a bad penny, poised for another jump over the precipice with an obsessive focus on finding ever more "biomarkers."

And, sad to say, there are many diseases where early detection, even if "biomarkers" are found, simply doesn't make any difference in the prognosis, management, or treatment of the disease. There are also many problems that may correct themselves over time due to the body's ability to heal itself without any need for dangerous tests, procedures, or treatments.

So, before you make your next doctor's appointment, be sure to consider the following very carefully. According to the American Board of Internal Medicine and National Physicians Alliance, these are the "top ten" most commonly performed tests you can actually omit:

1. **Annual physical exam:** On average for healthy adults, rather than detecting real problems, it is more likely to find

false positives or meaningless results leading to useless and dangerous procedures and/or more tests that lead nowhere.

2. **Annual EKG:** On average for people without heart disease, it is more likely to mislead than to find early problems–leading to further needless and dangerous tests, drugs, and even surgery.

3. **Annual "blood panel" tests:** For people who feel well in the first place, it is more likely to lead to false positives than to detect new disease.

4. **Annual cholesterol test:** If cholesterol previously tested "normal" (although what is considered normal is constantly being manipulated by industry- motivated NIH "reviews"), this test is needed only once every five years.

5. **Annual Pap Smear:** Although this is one very important and successful test for early detection of cervical cancer, it is only needed every three years in women who have tested normal.

6. **Prostate Specific Antigen (PSA) to detect prostate cancer:** Experts from the U.S. Preventative Services Task Force no longer recommend this test, saying it causes more harm than benefit. The harm is not from this test itself but that it is frequently misleading, resulting in useless procedures and surgery that frequently cause permanent disability or even death. Studies show that patients not given the PSA test have no higher mortality than patients faithfully screened for prostate cancer by this test.

7. **Pre-operative chest x-ray:** Many hospitals still require a routine chest x-ray prior to surgery but it is a wasted effort unless the patient has heart or lung disease. The annual routine chest x-ray as part of a yearly physical exam was given up long ago, since the risk from radiation far exceeded any benefit at detection of lung cancer. Of course, now you can give up the annual physical as well.

8. **Bone scans in women under 65 years:** Efforts to detect

osteoporosis in younger women have resulted in many women taking dangerous drugs with terrible side effects that are unnecessary (besides, if you wait until you're 65, Medicare will cover this test if medically necessary).

9. **Radiologic tests for low back pain:** If back pain is of short duration (less than 2–4 weeks), doing imaging studies add no benefit or improvement in outcome. And, as I've said before, the vast majority of patients with low back pain should be treated first with spinal manual therapy, provided by physical therapists and chiropractors, rather than drugs or surgery. And one hospital in Seattle is now doing just that with success (see below).

10. **Radiologic tests for headaches:** The common headache is sufficiently diagnosed by taking a careful medical history and doing a comprehensive neurological exam. Find a doctor who still knows how to provide that.

These 10 recommendations are not just theoretical. They are already being tried with positive results.

Local health care providers and some insurers are already improving the system by treating their patients better by providing less care. Following are just a few examples as reported in an editorial in *The New York Times* [76]

Premier Inc. is an alliance of hospitals around the country that has ceased doing useless blood tests and screenings. Over three years in 157 hospitals in 31 states they have saved almost 25,000 lives and reduced costs by almost $5 billion, saving 12 percent of their overall spending.

Virginia Mason Medical Center in Seattle stopped doing useless radiologic tests for headache and back pain, decreasing the use of CT scans by one-quarter. Also, in collaboration with Seattle-based Starbuck's and Aetna Insurance they stopped sending people with low back pain to expensive orthopedic specialists (who could only see them after lengthy and painful waits, and then order a costly

CT scan before providing any therapy). Instead they sent back pain patients directly for spinal manual therapy to physical therapists on the same day. Most patients were pain free and back to work in less time than it would have taken them to wait to see a medical specialist. And they avoided dangerous drugs and surgery.

That's true healthcare reform.

So what are the most common regular tests you should get?

They are actually few and simple.

For women over 40 it is useful to get a mammogram every two years.

After much controversy about the risks of mammograms, the optimal screening interval and hundreds of millions of dollars spent on research, the data indicate that it's simply not necessary to get a yearly mammogram. Bi-annually is just fine. However, women should perform frequent breast self-examinations (while standing in the shower or otherwise). Breast cancer remains the leading cancer among women, while heart disease is the leading cause of death overall (as in men).

So for heart disease, getting your blood pressure checked regularly is the single most important step you can take to prevent or control your risk. Unfortunately, as I reported in my *Daily Dispatch*, the healthcare system is failing miserably to detect and treat high blood pressure–which is an extremely treatable condition.

It's time to give up on all the dangerous and wasteful testing and focus on the things that really make a difference–and can literally mean the difference between life and death.

If your doctor is recommending any of the other 10 tests above, it can't hurt to talk to him candidly about the real risks and benefits. You can refer to the "Choose Wisely" campaign of the American Board of Internal Medicine Foundation. And of course, you can always get a second opinion. And if he doesn't recommend these tests, before you argue to have them just because everyone else is... you may want to consider counting your blessings. Instead, focus on what's really needed to ensure optimal health for whatever area of concern you may have.

Chapter 8
The deadly mammogram myth

Mammograms are one of those "routine" cancer screenings I mentioned in the previous chapter that affects millions of patients. Older women, in particular. And the dangers are very real.

Data shows mammograms do a lot less than you might think to save actual lives. And they have caused a sweeping epidemic of overdiagnosis and overtreatment. Yet, when you suggest anyone skip this cancer screening, or simply use it less frequently, politically correct zealots act as if you're mounting a campaign against women's health.

Of course, this reaction has very little to do with science. Indeed, when it comes to cancer–and breast cancer, in particular–politics, emotion, and fear can completely overwhelm the facts.

You see, 50 years ago, one clinical trial examined mammography as a screening tool for breast cancer. And in the ensuing years, legions of doctors, technicians, medical device makers, public health professionals, and government bureaucrats helped parlay this often-ineffective tool into a multi-billion-dollar enterprise.

Today, tens of millions of women dutifully get annual mammograms. They believe the mantra "early detection saves lives." But the real data about this approach shows otherwise...

In fact, doctors at the Geisel School of Medicine at Dartmouth University recently gave us some startlingly grim data about mammograms.[77]

According to their estimate, up to 3.2 women, but as few as 0.3 women, out of every 1,000 who get yearly mammograms over a decade will avoid dying of breast cancer. In other words, mammograms, at best, will save three out of every 1,000 women from dying of breast cancer over a decade. At worst, they will save no one.

But up to 67 percent of the women will have at least one false positive during those 10 years. Plus, for every 1,000 women screened over the decade, medical interventions will medically harm as many as 14 women with overdiagnosis and overtreatment.

Think about it this way…

According to this analysis, over a 10-year span, mammograms harm five times, and up to 50 times, as many women as they save. Plus, a majority of all these women will experience at least one traumatic "false-alarm" along the way.

Here's another problem with mammograms…

Aside from not preventing deaths any better than physical exams, they're also harmful. They may actually *increase* your risk of breast cancer by subjecting you to radiation–and by physically abusing breast tissue.

Over the past 25 years or so, the frequency of breast cancer has dramatically increased–from about 1 in 11 to now about 1 in 9 women. This past quarter-century is exactly the same time period of time that "everyone" has been getting mammograms.[78]

So maybe we are "detecting" more small cancers, and maybe even causing some, with annual mammograms. But remember, we're not lowering the death rates of the population.

Plus, mammograms are highly inaccurate. In fact, according to the National Institutes of Health, 90 percent of "abnormal" findings turn out to be false positives for breast cancer.

Even the pink-ribboned Komen Foundation admits when

Pass on the PSA, too

Like mammograms, the Prostate Specific Antigen (PSA) test to detect prostate cancer has been fraught with controversy In fact, experts from the U.S. Preventative Services Task Force no longer recommend this test, saying it causes more harm than benefit. The harm is not from this test itself but that it is frequently misleading, resulting in useless procedures and surgery that frequently cause permanent disability or even death. Studies show that patients not given the PSA test have no higher mortality than patients faithfully screened for prostate cancer by this test.

women get all the mammograms they recommend, 50 to 60 percent of them will end up with a false positive. So the majority of women get at least one traumatic "cancer scare" during their lifetime. (Ironically, mammograms miss 17 percent of breast cancers that <u>are</u> really present.)

Why all the false positives?

Well, today, mammograms are more sensitive than ever. They detect very small lesions of cells that look suspicious. So the woman (and her family) has to go through the pain and stress of a biopsy. But once you put the cells under a microscope, we discover they aren't cancerous at all.[79]

Even when we *do* classify these small lesions as "cancer," sometimes they *don't* really behave like cancer in the body. They will never cause illness or death. This is often true of ductal carcinomas of the breast. But they still get treated as real cancer. And we subject the women to the tortures and dangers of real cancer treatment.

In a recent interview with *Medscape* [80], my friend and colleague Dr. George Lundberg explained why it's important to assess each individual cancer carefully. He's the former editor-in-chief of the

Journal of the American Medical Association. He said:

> For a long time, it made sense to try to eradicate all cancers, as early and as completely as possible. Mass efforts were launched to find cancers wherever they were and destroy them. Since the earliest cancers seemed to evolve from some identifiable premalignant conditions, wouldn't it make sense to also nip those in the bud? Sounds logical.

> But, as with many exuberant efforts, this one got out of control. Many lesions that were called "cancer" really were not cancers at all in behavior, and this fact began to be recognized in large numbers of patients. These unfortunate victims have experienced massive psychological and physical harm and costs without any clear benefits achieved by finding and treating their "non-cancers."

> And here's the real kicker...

> In the cases where a woman has a real, aggressive cancer, and the mammogram finds it, she still needs a biopsy. And that biopsy can end up spreading the cancer.

> Overall, mammograms are ineffective for the population as a whole. And sometimes dangerous. They also contribute to the epidemic of over-diagnosis and over-treatment of cancers. This has helped feed the growing beast of today's cancer industry.

> Having said all of this, there are of course individual examples of women who discover they have breast cancer through their annual mammogram. Presumably, they would not have found it otherwise. Ultimately, the early detection made a real difference in their treatment and survival. But, of course, we will never know what *would* have happened in any individual case if she had not gotten that mammogram. That's why we do research to learn more about the real benefits of early cancer detection.

> As a reminder, these *real* risk factors for breast cancer are:
> - Early age at menarche (early puberty)
> - Late age at menopause

- Having few (or no) pregnancies
- Late age at first pregnancy (over 30 years old)
- Lack of breastfeeding
- Lack of being breastfed (as an infant)
- Taking certain birth control and hormone drugs
- Having one or more first degree relatives with breast cancer
- Genetic risk according to the "BRAC" gene test

Of course every woman is an individual. With individual risk and concerns. So–what are your options as an individual?

First, always consult with your trusted, qualified doctor to make a personalized plan. Look at whether you have any of the real risk factors for breast cancer I've mentioned above.

Secondly, consider thermography. It's an alternative screening test that uses no painful mechanical pressure or dangerous radiation. It's a form of thermal (infrared) imaging, so it doesn't damage the sensitive breast tissue as mammograms can. Plus, studies show it identifies precancerous or cancerous cells earlier. And it produces clear results, which cuts down on additional testing.

While mammograms do still have a role in the world of cancer screening (albeit a smaller, less frequent role than currently used by the mainstream), in the next chapter, I'll tell you about one common method of cancer screening that should really be eliminated altogether in favor of safer, simpler alternatives.

Chapter 9

The hidden, grisly dangers of "routine" colonoscopies

The U.S. is well-known for its massive expenditures on end-of-life care. On average, people here incur more medical costs during the last six months of life than during their entire life up until then. But it turns out the cost of ordinary care is nothing to sneeze at either.

"Routine" tests and exams add up to $2.7 trillion per year (even more than the federal government's annual deficit).[81] Colonoscopies are a case in point.

Colonoscopy is—by far—the most expensive screening test that Americans are exhorted to undergo. But there are several reasons you should think twice before "bending over," when it comes again. In fact, skipping your next routine colonoscopy might actually save your life.

There are some serious dangers associated with this supposedly safe test you won't hear about from the public health "experts." Or the mainstream hype. There are also alternatives to colonoscopy that are just as effective—and much safer (not to mention less expensive). More on that in just a moment. But first, let me tell you why some real health experts are questioning whether it's truly worth it to get a colonoscopy once you hit a certain age...

"Too old" for a colonoscopy?

The minute you hit 50, your doctor probably started encouraging you to get regular colonoscopies.

But at this point in life, is a colonoscopy really worth it?

You see, the major purpose of routine colonoscopies is to detect polyps growing from the mucosal surface of the colon. But it takes, on average, 15 years for cancer within a polyp to develop into full-blown colon cancer.[82]

Yes, some people have a specific genetic predisposition which can lead to multiple polyps and a higher risk of colon cancer. And these people should be followed and managed closely. But anyone can potentially develop a colon polyp. And in light of that 15-year lag time, how old is "too old" to go through this uncomfortable procedure and be subjected to its risks? This question is important because "routine" colonoscopy can be quite dangerous—even fatal.

Horror-film injuries from a "routine" test

Colonoscopy is portrayed as a benign, safe procedure for everyone. But in my forensic medicine practice I have seen case after case of perforated intestines and peritonitis (a potentially fatal inflammation of the abdominal lining), lacerated and punctured livers with massive bleeding, and other fatal complications. All from "routine" colonoscopies.

I even had one case in which the air pumped into the colon (to inflate it for easy examination) escaped into the patient's abdominal cavity. It put so much pressure on the liver that it cut off blood supply back to the heart. The patient died from shock.

To make matters worse, colonoscopies are often prescribed more frequently than medical guidelines recommend.

ACOG in the wheel

Ten years ago, apparently having run out of things to say on TV from one end, Katie Couric had her colonoscopy performed on the other end, live, on national TV. Patients began demanding them like the latest cosmetic procedure. Then, the American College of Gastroenterology (ACOG) successfully lobbied Congress to have the procedure covered by Medicare (in other words, us, the taxpayers).

So now, when you become eligible for Medicare at age 65, with the 15 year lag time for a polyp to become cancerous, this Medicare benefit can help you avoid coming down with colon cancer at age 80 years or older, on average. Just doing the math. But I digress...

The fact is, several much less expensive and less dangerous techniques are also effective. Yet specialist medical practitioners have (not surprisingly) picked the most expensive—and dangerous—option. Without any scientific data to support it. I know it sounds bizarre, given all the hype and increased recommendations for colonoscopy...but it's true.

In fact, according to a study published earlier this year in the *American Journal of Gastroenterology*, colonoscopy has never even been compared to other, much safer—and less expensive—screening methods head-to-head in randomized trials. This despite the continual call from mainstream medicine for ever more randomized, controlled, clinical trials—which are considered the "gold standard."

Until the last 10-15 years, colonoscopies were only performed in doctor's offices. And only on patients at high risk for colon cancer or who were experiencing intestinal bleeding.

Then doctors reported they could detect early cancers even in people who are not at high risk and don't have bleeding. But, according to an article published in the Journal of the *National Cancer Institute*, there is no compelling evidence that colonoscopy offers any additional benefit over the older, cheaper, safer tests.[83]

And the bottom line is <u>no study has shown that colonoscopy prevents colon cancer incidence or mortality any more than the other safer, less expensive screening methods</u>.

Nonetheless, the ACOG unilaterally declared colonoscopy as the "preferred" approach to colon cancer prevention. It certainly was preferred when it came to collecting membership dues apparently.

Of course, colonoscopy has also become very lucrative. One analysis even reported colonoscopy is <u>the</u> reason the U.S. leads the world in health expenditures!

But some primary care doctors don't realize the costs of the tests and procedures they prescribe.

The most expensive hour you'll ever spend

A colleague of mine in Hartford, CT recently called the local hospital in order to price a colonoscopy. And even he couldn't get an answer.

Because this "routine" screening procedure can cost anywhere from $6,000 to nearly $20,000. For an outpatient procedure requiring less than an hour.

They are the most expensive screening tests that otherwise healthy Americans undergo. In fact, colonoscopies in the U.S. often cost more than childbirth or an appendectomy in most other developed countries.[84]

But colonoscopies represent such a large financial burden because, unlike hip replacements, c-sections, or even nose spray, everybody gets them—or is supposed to, whether they need it or not.

The final "knock-out" blow

And on top of all this, there is the "wild west" of administering anesthesia during colonoscopies. Not only does anesthesia add to the procedure's risk, but this service is billed separately—and is all over the map.

For anesthesia during one surgical procedure, for the exact same service, one anesthesia group practice charges $6,970 from a large private health insurer, $5,208 from Blue Cross Blue Shield, $1,605 from Medicare, and $797 from Medicaid.[85] *What* is the real cost of providing this service? Who knows!

A better question is: *Why* are anesthesiologists involved in colonoscopies at all?

Colonoscopy does not require general anesthesia. Moderate sedation—a drug like Valium, or another intravenous medicine that takes effect and wears off quickly—is all you really need. Both of which could technically be administered by any nurse in any doctor's office. There is <u>no clinical benefit</u> whatsoever from having anesthesiologists involved in this procedure. But it adds a further cost of $1.1 billon per year.[86, 87]

So, who is keeping the anesthesiologists where they don't belong? Our "friends" at the FDA. They refuse to modify the drug <u>labels</u> advising that moderate sedation must be performed in the presence of an anesthesiologist (a policy that the American Society of Anesthesiologists lobbies strongly to keep in place, of course).

So all of this leads us to the $1 billion question…

What are the alternatives?

Here we have yet another situation where the most expensive, most dangerous screening procedure has simply never been proven to be better than less expensive, safer procedures.

Three proven alternatives to colonoscopy are:

1. The long-established **hemoccult test** detects blood in the stool as a sign of intestinal bleeding. When there is bleeding in the lower intestinal tract it can be seen as bright red blood in the stool. But when the bleeding is higher up, the blood breaks down and becomes invisible, or "occult." Fecal occult blood testing can decrease the risk of death from colorectal cancer by 33 percent.[88] Not bad for a test that is cheap, and completely safe, non-invasive, and that you can administer yourself in the privacy of your own bathroom.

2. To get an actual look inside the lower intestine, opt for a **sigmoidoscopy**. Unlike colonoscopy, which examines the entire colon, sigmoidoscopy only enters the lower large intestine, which is where most cancers occur. Several recent studies have shown that this screening method is as effective as colonoscopy—if not more so.[89, 90] In fact, according to one of these studies, getting just ONE sigmoidoscopy between

the ages of 55-64 can reduce incidence of colon cancer by 31 percent and colon cancer mortality by 38 percent.[91] A sigmoidoscopy can be done right in your doctor's office and doesn't require any sedation. Which makes it much less expensive—and also much safer—than colonoscopy.

3. A relatively recent development has been CT colonography, which involves doing CT scans to detect colon polyps. In general, CT colonography is done every five years, but radiologists have worked out several more specific guidelines for individual cases (including instances of positive fecal occult blood tests (FOBT), and to deal with the frequent problem of an "incomplete colonoscopy.")

Please don't misunderstand my intention. In no way am I downplaying the importance of colon cancer and effective screening for this potentially deadly disease. However, I and many others do take issue with the medical subspecialist's carte blanche recommendation of colonoscopy. The available science simply doesn't support it as the be-all, end-all of colon cancer screening. And, as always, when it comes to your health, it's absolutely critical to follow the science.

The fact is, there are serious risks associated with colonoscopy… and its superiority is unproven. But there ARE alternatives. Safer ones. That do a better (or, at the very least, safer) job of reducing mortality from this disease.

If you have your doubts about getting a colonoscopy, make sure to consult with your primary care physician regarding your family history, personal medical history, and any current health problems or symptoms, to find out whether starting with safer, less expensive options—a hemoccult test, a sigmoidoscopy, or the new CT colonography scan—may be right for you for colon cancer screening and prevention.

And remember, you can lower your risk of colon cancer in the first place (and any other form of cancer, as well as many other chronic diseases, for that matter) by following the diet, exercise, and supplement recommendations you'll find throughout your issues of Insiders' Cures.

* * * *

There is more to consider when it comes to fighting cancer. You've read about some heavy-hitters here, but there are many other specific nutrients, plant compounds, as well as mind-body therapies that when combined can have added benefit. You can find most of these products on your own—most now readily available at health food stores, and some of the more basic even at the grocery store and natural food stores.

If you want to help lower your risk for developing cancer you can use good quality supplements on your own following these guidelines. If you are suffering from cancer, or recovering from cancer or the toxic effects of mainstream cancer therapy, work with a qualified practitioner to find the approaches that are right for you. Beyond diet, nutrition, and dietary supplements, mind-body therapies are very effect for cancer patients and cancer survivors as true complementary medicine. An important step is to determine which mind-body therapies will work for you, and it is important to learn your "emotional type" by taking my simple survey in my book with Mike Jawer, *Your Emotional Type* (available through www. DrMicozzi.com or at your local bookstore).

If you have cancer or are a cancer survivor, don't try to conquer cancer on your own. It requires support from friends, family, and knowledgeable health practitioners.

For more detailed information on complementary approaches to cancer, see my 700-page handbook geared toward practitioners, *Complementary & Integrative Medicine in Cancer Care and Prevention*, New York: Springer, 2007.

Another new way to avoid costly, dangerous colonoscopies

This alternative to colonoscopies became available in November of 2014. And it's a boon to millions of people who prefer to avoid the discomfort, danger and expense of colonoscopies–and instead want to do their own colon cancer screening at home. The new test makes use of one of the long-awaited promises of biotech. It's the first to detect cancer-related DNA in stool. You can't get more precise than that.

This home procedure is a reliable test that doesn't require the painful preparations that interfere with your life. Nor does it carry the dangerous risks and awful complications that may cost you your life. There's no tortuous "prep," no scope, no anesthesia–and no risk to the procedure.

But, of course, the threatened colonoscopy industry is already trying to dump on this new test. They admit this simple, safe test will boost effective screening for colon cancer. But then they try to claim that it will lure people away from colonoscopies, which they say have been "shown" to save lives.

This test will certainly "lure" people away from the costs and disastrous consequences of colonoscopies. And it will certainly make it easier, safer and more palatable for more people to get effective screening for colon cancer.

But hold on–the dodgy claim that colonoscopies are better at "saving lives" has never been proven.

The fact is, we don't have any head-to-head, controlled clinical trial comparisons of using colonoscopy vs. alternatives test like the old standby fecal occult blood test or FIT (fecal immunochemical test). And there are no comparisons for the new test.

Even the National Cancer Institute (NCI) experts say the new test looks promising. (And this organization, as you'll recall, derided the new lung cancer screening test, largely based, as far as I can tell, on unethical and unscientific bias against lung cancer victims. Although the U.S. Centers for *Medicare* and Medicaid Services (*CMS*) finally just approved it for coverage under Medicare.)

The FDA approved the new colon cancer screening test in September 2014. And the world-respected Mayo Clinic, where it was developed, now offers the test. Exact Sciences Corp of Madison, WI will sell it under the name Cologuard®. And the Mayo Clinic will get royalties. (So it does not exactly sound like another big pharma venture.)

The idea and procedure itself are simple.

Patients obtain and send a stool sample to the lab where the test detects any blood (like the old home tests). The presence of blood could indicate the presence of a tumor. Plus, Cologuard detects the presence of mutated DNA, which could signal cancer or a precancerous growth called a polyp.

If the test is positive for cancer, then the patient undertakes additional diagnostic steps, such as a colonoscopy or sigmoidoscopy, to remove the growth or polyp. Sigmoidoscopy, which looks at the lower portion of the colon (where cancers most commonly occur) is a safer option and doesn't require sedation. In Europe, sigmoidoscopy is virtually the only "scoping" done.

Of course, the only real measure of the worth of any cancer screening procedure is whether it lowers the risk of cancer death. (As I have pointed out before, use of mainstream government-industrial-medical approaches to screening breast, prostate, and colon cancer have yet to specifically show to any clear benefits in actually reducing cancer death rates in the overall population.)

But this new Cologuard test *does* appear to lower the risk of cancer death...

In a large study, researchers compared Cologuard to one of the older tests for fecal blood. The Cologuard test detected 92 percent of colorectal cancers and 42 percent of precancerous growths (polyps). By comparison, the older fecal blood test only detected 74 percent of cancers and 24 percent of polyps.

Like any test, the increased sensitivity of Cologuard at detecting real cancers also leads to more false positives. In other words, the test can sometimes find evidence of a polyp or cancer where none is present. And it correctly rules out cancer 87 percent of the time (compared to 95 percent for the older blood test).

Critics complain this means 13 percent of patients may go on to get colonoscopies anyway who don't really need them. But, let's stop and think logically about this point for a moment. Do they really think it's better to make 100 percent of patients get colonoscopies whether they need them or not…or just 13 percent of them who really do need them?

Cologuard can avoid the costs, risks, and problems of colonoscopy 87 percent of the time. And that's a huge accomplishment.

Medicare jointly reviewed the Cologuard test with the FDA. (It was a rare example of sensible, federal bureaucratic coordination.) It will also pay for the test for Medicare patients, so the $599 cost should not be a barrier (especially when compared to the bloated costs of colonoscopies).

Now, keep these two things in mind…

First–it takes 15 years, on average, for a precancerous polyp to became a cancer. So there is time and opportunity to catch it with regular, non-invasive testing.

Second–you don't need any fancy test to detect rectal growths. Government statisticians certainly like to lump all "colo-rectal" cancers together to make their "survival" rates look better. But colon cancer is very different from rectal cancer. And doctors can easily detect rectal growths, polyps and cancers with the old fashioned, digital rectal exam, as part of a routine physical examination. (If doctors are given enough time to do it anymore, that is.)

All statistics aside, sensible cancer experts say the best colon cancer screening test is one that people will actually go and get. So if the torturous colonoscopy prep turns you off, ask your doctor about this new Cologuard test. It's yet another good alternative to dangerous colonoscopies

HEALING PAIN INSTEAD OF TREATING PAIN

Part 2: Healing pain instead of treating pain

Chapter 10
The great evolutionary trade-off

I always stress the importance of your gait (or how well you walk) as a key to health and longevity, especially as you get older. But it's not about *how much you walk*. It's about *how well you walk*. And indeed, it's the ability to walk upright that sets humans apart—but it's also what sets up for a lot of pain as well.

Walking has been a key factor in the ability of humans to survive. In fact, the ability to walk upright on two legs is a distinctly human trait. And throughout human history, this trait has freed the hands so that, together with larger brains, humans could express their creativity and productivity to build our modern, "man-made" world.

One important trade-off is that in order to walk (and run) more effectively, the legs needed to be placed more narrowly together than they are on other, four-footed mammals. This effect results in a narrower pelvis, especially at the hips.

However, humans have developed very large brains. So women need to have wider hips to allow infants to pass safely through the birth canal. (*Interesting side note:* Humans are the only animals who have such potentially difficult delivery, which is why we call it "labor.")

But since you can't walk effectively if the hips are <u>too</u> wide, human infants were born at earlier and earlier stages of development, while the brain is still immature. So human young are the most immature creatures in the universe, and require a prolonged period of dependency—with implications for nuclear family, extended family, post-reproductive grandparents, and human social organization as a whole.

Consider it a grand evolutionary biological compromise between upright posture, freeing the hands, and having bigger brains.

But there's another tremendous impact that walking upright has had on humans. One that millions of people struggle with every day—back pain.

From discomfort to disability

The spine provides structure to the entire body and helps protect the vital organs. It also provides the protective conduit for the "wiring" that runs to all the parts of the body—the spinal cord and the spinal nerves.

In animals that walk on all fours, the natural design of the spine is like a simple suspension bridge. But over time (millions of years, probably), humans began to stand erect. And the shape of the spine converted from a suspension bridge to a shallow S-shaped (or sigmoid) curve...to provide balance, structural support, and some "suspension" as well as "shock absorption."

But as you can imagine, pounding away against hard surfaces while walking not only affects the joints of the legs, but the shock waves work their way up through the pelvis to the spinal column and the individual vertebrae. The result is degenerative arthritis, or osteoarthritis in the spine.

And just like in other joints, osteoarthritis of the spinal vertebrae can lead to stiffness. As well as contribute to bony outgrowths that can impact and irritate the spinal nerves that branch out from the spinal cord. These kinds of irritations are common in the arms and the legs ("pinched nerves"). And on a chronic basis, they can cause the familiar condition of "sciatica."

In the spine itself, the middle 12 vertebra are held relatively rigid by the ribs, but the seven cervical vertebrae in the neck, and the five lumbar vertebrae of the lower back have more degrees of freedom, and less support. Which is why lower back pain is such a universal source of discomfort in humans.

Of course, when there is a sudden rupture of a spinal disc (or cushion), or even a traumatic fracture of a portion of a vertebra, there can be sudden debilitating pain.

However, even without a sudden rupture or traumatic fracture, low back pain can be disabling. In fact, it's the most common cause of disability in working Americans (those who still have work).

Why back surgery should be your last resort

Low back pain may be an unavoidable consequence of walking upright. But living with it doesn't need to be.

And there are treatments for back pain that are much safer—not to mention more effective—than dangerous painkilling drugs and potentially disastrous back surgery.

In fact, surgery should be your absolute last resort. The results can be debilitating. And there's no "going back" from surgery.

Back surgery has become such a problem that is has actually spawned a new medical condition, called "failed back" syndrome. And there are doctors who specialize in treating people with it. It's become a kind of "crisis." But as I said to Pennsylvania Governor Ed Rendell at a U.S. Congressional Field Hearing in Pennsylvania in February 2003, perhaps this crisis is a blessing in disguise. Because it should finally help open the door for the effective, non-surgical treatments that can help the vast majority of people with back pain.

To his great credit (on this and many other public policy issues), Governor Rendell was genuinely concerned and refreshingly open-minded. And a few weeks later, he contacted me to provide all the details on these alternatives to his office in Harrisburg.

That information included overwhelming evidence about one particular—and *completely non-invasive*—treatment that works for almost every person who tries it...

Surgery-free pain relief

Spinal manual therapy (SMT), is the most effective and cost-effective treatment for most patients with low back pain. SMT is a technique for adjusting the alignment of the spinal vertebrae and other joints. Many believe that in addition to aligning the body adjustment balances the energy flow through the body similar to the concepts of many Asian medical therapies. SMT is the primary treatment provided by chiropractors.

Chiropractors have historically emphasized the intimate relations in the body between **structure and function**, the mediating role of the **nervous system**, and the need for restoration and maintenance of structural and functional **balance** of the spine and musculoskeletal system. From this perspective, balance is the key—and the presence or absence of pain is incidental. For patients, however, pain is almost always the primary concern.

In recent years, the mainstreaming of chiropractic has taken many forms. Low back guidelines from government agencies in the United States, Great Britain, Australia, New Zealand, Denmark and Sweden have recognized spinal manipulation as one of a very small number of effective treatment methods for lower back pain.

In fact, a decade ago the former U.S. Agency for Health Care Policy & Research conducted a review and found SMT to be the most safe and effective treatment. Unlike the NIH, this agency was focused on using research and science to help guide rational medical practices. Things that would actually benefit the public.

Of course, their recommendation for SMT outraged orthopedic surgeons. So much so that they attempted to have the agency shut down. When that didn't work, they tried to have it de-funded. Eventually, they managed to at least get the office reorganized. (Today it's known as the Agency for Health Care Quality, and has little power to actually influence medical practice compared to the "medical mandarins" at NIH, or the federal purse strings controlled by Health Care Finance Administration and the Center for Medicare and Medicaid Services.)

But I digress...

At about this same time—during 2002-2003—I received a

grant from the US Health Resources and Services Administration (another rare honest broker) to review all the studies on low back pain that had been done worldwide.

I worked with the Palmer College Research Consortium and a dozen other universities and scores of scientists around the country. And found—no matter how you sliced it—that spinal manual therapy (SMT) is indeed a safe and effective treatment for low back pain.

And, even better—it's easy to access. There are over 50,000 practicing chiropractors in the US (all of them from accredited schools). They are licensed in every state. But if you can't find a chiropractor near you for some reason, physical therapists also provide effective SMT.

Other useful therapies for low back pain include massage and acupuncture. But with the overwhelming evidence for and easy availability of SMT, most people should try it first.

Chapter 11

The problem with pain:
Another reason the government is literally
a pain in the neck...and back, and head, etc.

In the history of American medicine, alleviating pain has been one of the two central tenants of "rational medicine." (Preventing death was the other). Unfortunately, there's nothing rational about the way mainstream medicine handles pain relief these days.

From the arid mountains of Afghanistan, to the jungles of Honduras, from the gritty urban streets of New York, to the fruited plains of Nebraska, the government is hard at work protecting you from pain...medications.

You see, we live in an era where another misguided government "war"—this one on drugs—is intimidating competent and honest doctors and nurses. Keeping them from prescribing and administering adequate pain medication in effective doses. Even for those on their deathbeds, who often must suffer their last moments on earth in debilitating pain.

All under the guise of "protecting" the public from becoming addicted to pain killers.

If the situation sounds bleak, well…in many ways, it is. But before you give up hope, there is good news.

The fact is, there are many alternatives that can offer you *real relief*. For just about any type of pain. Ones you won't hear about from the government medical bureaucracy. (Whose agenda has nothing to do with actually helping those who are suffering.)

So let me tell you a bit about why the "War on Drugs" has turned into a "War on People in Pain."

The best painkiller on earth that the government is desperate to keep out of your hands

Despite its potential for misuse, the opium poppy (*Papaver somniferum*) has been one of nature's best gifts to humankind. It is, without a doubt, the world's most effective pain medicine. Opium is the source of morphine and all its various modern derivatives.

And to this day, even in our era of modern pharmaceuticals, morphine and morphine derivatives still have unmatched pain relieving and other healing properties. And they remain in widespread use throughout the world.

The reason they're so effective is that our brains and central nervous systems have built-in receptors for the opiates in these medications. It's a match made in pain-relief heaven.

But, unfortunately, like many good things, opium also has a history of abuse. And that's where the focus has been for centuries.

So although morphine, hydromorphone, oxycodone, and codeine remain the gold standard opioid analgesics, the ham-fisted prosecution of drug wars has made many good doctors afraid to prescribe them. And as a result, the pharmaceutical industry has put out a slew of rival analgesics. These rival pain meds are less restricted than the opioids. The problem is, they're also typically less effective. And more toxic.

53 years of useless—and dangerous— "relief"

For example, until recently, roughly 10 million Americans were taking the painkilling drug propoxyphene (sold as Darvon and Darvocet). But in November 2010, the FDA pulled it from the market because of serious heart risks. But here's the really interesting part of the Darvon story…

While it is classified by the DEA and FDA as a narcotic, it has never been shown in controlled studies to be even a **weak** analgesic.

In other words, it has all of the stimulating, addictive effects of opioids. But *none* of the pain-relieving benefits. Yet the FDA approved it for that very use back in the 1950s. Putting millions of people at risk for addiction, heart complications, and who knows what else for 53 years. Risk with absolutely no "reward" in the form of relief.

Then, to add insult to injury, the FDA recommended doctors switch patients to other painkillers, notably Extra Strength Tylenol (acetaminophen).

Take that advice and you trade in risk of heart problems for liver failure.

That's right. This common, over-the-counter painkiller—found in nearly every medicine cabinet in America—causes hundreds of deaths each year due to liver toxicity. But until now (there was finally a class action suit filed in 2012) nobody talked about it.

It's yet another example of major medical mismanagement spawned by ill-informed politicians and misbegotten government regulatory agencies.

But, again, just because the government denies citizens access to one form of effective pain relief doesn't mean you have to suffer. In fact, there are many other effective, natural options for alleviating pain.

The whole-body approach to pain relief

Conventional medicine is always focused on suppressing symptoms. And it frequently assumes that the location of pain is also the site of its cause and origin. Thus, knee pain is generally assumed to be a knee problem, shoulder pain is assumed to be a shoulder problem, and so forth.

This pain-centered diagnostic logic frequently leads to increasingly sophisticated and invasive diagnostic and therapeutic procedures. For example, if physical examination of the knee fails to define the problem clearly, the knee is x-rayed. If the x-ray film fails to offer adequate clarification, magnetic resonance imaging (MRI) of the knee is performed, and in some cases a surgical procedure follows. All the while, this search for knee pain may be missing the obvious fact that the pain is caused by misalignment of the hip at the pelvis.

We should all remember the song from our childhood: "The knee bone's connected to the hip bone, the hip bone's connected to the back bone...."

The chiropractic approach to musculoskeletal pain involves evaluating the site of pain in a both regional and whole-body context. Although shoulder, elbow, and wrist problems can be caused by injuries or pathologies in these areas, pain in and around each of the shoulder, elbow, and wrist joints can also have as its source segmental dysfunction (subluxation) in the cervical spine.

Similarly, symptoms in the hip, knee, and ankle can also originate at the site of the pain, but in many cases the source lies in the lumbar spine or sacroiliac joints. Pain in the knee might come from the knee itself, but tracing the nerve pathways between the knee and the spine reveals possible areas of causation in and around the hip, in the deep muscles of the buttocks or pelvis, in the sacroiliac joints, or in the lumbar spine.

Of course, chiropractors also use diagnostic tools such as radiography and MRI. The point isn't to disregard these technologies completely, but to present an alternative diagnostic model.

After all, it happens all too frequently where a patient undergoes this entire high-tech diagnostic scenario. After suffering through it waiting for a "diagnosis," the poor patient finally stumbles into the chiropractor (if he or she can still walk!). And finally, his or her knee problem is discovered to be a compensation for a mechanical disorder in the lower back. Of course, even despite months of needless suffering, patients are still fortunate if they find the chiropractor before they agree to surgery.

The point here is that chiropractic SMT can provide effective relief even for pain that doesn't seem to have anything to do with your back or spine. Research shows it can be effective for neck pain, leg pain, headaches, and more.

Three herbal pain soothers worth a try

While they're not a substitute for effective spinal manual therapies, there are several herbs that can help relieve pain. They include:

- Boswellia serratta extract (gum)—400 -500 mg/day
- Curcuma longa (root) (Tumeric)—200 mg/day
- Withania somnifera (root extract) (Ashwaganda)—500 mg/day

Chapter 12
Managing migraines without drugs

Headache is probably the single most common cause of pain experienced regularly by most people. And the most difficult type of headache to treat is the migraine. But, again, there are very effective natural treatments. Ones that can actually keep migraines from occurring in the first place. And if you've ever had a migraine, you know that an ounce of prevention is definitely worth a pound of cure. But before I get to the natural solutions for treating and preventing migraines, let's back up a step and talk about the onset of these often-debilitating headaches.

Too quick to pull the migraine trigger?

If you suffer from migraines, you may think chocolate or bright lights trigger your headaches. So you avoid these triggers at all costs. But that cause-and-effect relationship may not be as strong as you think.

In fact, Dutch scientists recently took a close look at two classic migraine triggers: exercise and bright light. The scientists wanted to know if exposure to classic triggers always results in migraine attacks. And are migraine "triggers" as strong as patients believe?

For the study, a team of researchers led by Anders Hougaard, M.D. recruited 27 migraine sufferers.[1] Each of the patients said that bright or flickering lights or strenuous activity triggered their migraines. So, the researchers tried to *provoke* migraines in the patients using these reported triggers.

They exposed the patients to bright lights, strenuous activity, or a combination of both triggers. Only three patients (11 percent) actually had migraine attacks with aura following these provocative tests. Three other patients reported migraines but without aura. The researchers discovered that exercise proved a stronger trigger than light exposure.

Dr. Hougaard suggested that these results could benefit migraine patients. "Migraine patients are usually advised to identify triggers and try and avoid them," he told *Medscape Medical News*.[2] "But our research suggests that this may be limiting people's lives and causing unnecessary stress in trying to avoid a wide range of factors which may turn out not to be triggers after all."

In fact, Dr. Hougaard warns migraine patients to carefully evaluate whether or not something is an actual trigger. He said, "Patients need to try to identify triggers but they need to establish that they are true triggers before cutting them out of their lives. So I would advise that they allow several exposures before defining a trigger."

So if you suffer from migraines, be very careful before you blindly cut out all "classic" triggers. Especially since many purported triggers—such as sunlight, exercise, wine, coffee, chocolate, and cheese—are actually *good* for you in moderation!

Plus, many other factors affect your threshold for a migraine attack. In fact, your fatigue, your hormone levels, and even the time of day can make you more vulnerable to an attack. For instance, how tired were you when you drank that glass of wine? Or were certain hormones high when you went for that three-mile run in the bright morning light?

In addition, you may confuse migraine "triggers" with cravings or certain behaviors. We know that feelings of tiredness, excitement, and depression, or food cravings often *precede* migraines. So, you may think eating chocolate triggers the migraine. But it's really a warning signal. Doctors call it a "premonitory symptom."

For example, you may crave chocolate one afternoon, so you eat a small piece of a candy bar. By dinnertime, you have a migraine. You kick yourself and think the chocolate triggered the migraine. But chocolate wasn't really the trigger. The craving was actually part of the onset of the migraine itself.

My former colleague, Stephen D. Silberstein, M.D., is a Professor of Neurology and Director of the headache center at Thomas Jefferson University. He agrees that avoiding triggers may be flawed advice. He says, "If migraine is a disorder of habituation of the brain to ordinary sensory signals, should one try to train the brain to habituate rather than avoid the trigger?"

That may explain why biofeedback helps so many migraine sufferers. With biofeedback, you learn to control your body's functions. You watch or listen to a monitor. And you learn by trial and error to control your heart rate, temperature, even your brain wave patterns. With biofeedback, can you may even be able to train your brain to handle exposure to so-called triggers, as my colleague suggests.

If you suffer from migraines, I recommend investigating biofeedback along with other "mind-body" therapies. You should choose these therapies based on your emotional "type." I explain all about this in my book *Your Emotional Type*.

But there are several other natural ways to manage migraines in addition to biofeedback.

Feverfew is probably the most well-known natural migraine remedy. This herb is a short, bushy flowering plant that grows in fields and along roadsides and blooms from July to October. The leaves have been used for all sorts of medicinal purposes since the ancient Greek and Roman physicians. Recently, though, it was approved for treating migraine headaches in both the United Kingdom and Canada.

A dried feverfew leaf preparation containing a minimum of 0.2% parthenolide (the active ingredient) is effective for preventing migraines. You'll need at least 125 mg per day.

Although it's most commonly used to improve cognitive function, **Ginkgo biloba** may also help ward off migraines. The effective dose is 120-240 mg per day.

And anyone who experiences regular migraines should be taking 200-600 milligrams of magnesium per day. Low levels of *magnesium* can contribute to migraines.

Food allergy may also be a problem for some migraine sufferers. The most common allergens (in decreasing order) include wheat (gluten), orange, egg, coffee/tea, milk, chocolate, corn, sugar, yeast, mushrooms, and peas. A small proportion of migraine sufferers may also react to the presence of tyramine in foods such as aged cheeses, yogurt, beer, wine, liver and organ meats.

If you use the above remedies and for some reason still find yourself battling a migraine at some point, there are a couple of reports that ginger may help them go away sooner. Mix 500-600 mg ginger powder with water and drink it every 4 hours until the migraine subsides (for up to four days—but hopefully not that long!).

Another, lesser-known herb—**butterbur**—made history in 2012 by gaining recognition from the American Academy of Neurology (AAN) as an effective migraine therapy.

In 2012, the AAN reviewed all the studies for alternative migraine treatments published between June 1999 and May 2007. Butterbur (*Petasites hybridis*) stood out as an effective alternative to prescription drugs. And, given all the clinical research on butterbur, the AAN's announcement is well-deserved.[3]

Several clinical trials published over the last 10 years prove that butterbur can help patients who get migraines on a regular basis. In fact, in many of these trials, patients who took butterbur root extract reduced the frequency of their migraines by up to 50 percent.[4]

Beyond butterbur extracts, experts reviewed other alternatives such as Co-enzyme Q10, magnesium, and hyperbaric oxygen as treatments. In addition, they reviewed Papaverine (a derivative of the opium poppy, Papaver somniferum). Papaverine affects blood circulation in the brain, which is a key factor in migraine headaches. Not surprisingly, Papaverine also works extremely well as a pain reliever.

In the AAN report, the neurologists acknowledged that non-prescription drugs are important for many migraine patients.

This is a big step for the AAN. It's important to migraine sufferers too because standard migraine drugs can cause serious side effects. And, in too many cases, the drugs just don't help! In fact, in severe cases, the very drugs prescribed to treat the migraine can *lead to chronic, unremitting headaches that never go away.*

But the good news is, there are many healthy alternatives to help!

Chapter 13

Why those tired, old natural arthritis "fixes" don't work
Plus, the long-forgotten ancient remedies that DO

Far too many people think glucosamine and chondroitin are a one-stop solution to arthritis pain.

If glucosamine and chondroitin were truly the wonder nutrient supplements that marketers claim they are, we wouldn't still be talking about arthritis. In fact, with all the "solutions" that have been dumped onto the public for decades, joint pain should have gone the way of the dinosaurs years ago.

Yet, as long as there have been joints, there has been joint pain.

Historians tell us that, unlike many common diseases that have become more prevalent in our modern industrialized era (think cancer and heart disease), arthritis has been afflicting humans since prehistoric times. In fact, paleopathologists estimate almost half of early humans—as far back as Neanderthal man—suffered some sort of joint condition.

Unfortunately, the best- documented health problem in human history is plaguing us still. And it will for generations to come—if we keep putting faith in supplements that get it all wrong.

But the good news is when an ailment has this much history, we have the benefit of millennia of trial and error before us. And our ancestors—from many cultures around the world—have left us clues that point us to real solutions for joint pain.

I've spent years investigating history's clues, and I've found alternatives to glucosamine and chondroitin that actually work. So let's get down to the real cause of this problem first.

The REAL cause of joint pain is something glucosamine can't touch

Joint pain fits into one of four categories:

1. Osteoarthritis. Deterioration from "wear-and-tear" on joints that leads to painful inflammation.

2. Rheumatoid arthritis. The immune system itself attacks joints, causing pain and deterioration. (More on this in Chapter 14.)

3. Degeneration of the discs. The discs between the vertebrae in the spine wear down, causing neck and back pain. (See Chapter 10 for more on back pain.)

4. Pains of undetermined nature. These may be linked to mind-body-immune system connections, as explained in my book with Mike Jawer, *Your Emotional Type* (www.drmicozzi. com).

But while there are different types of joint pain, they ultimately have one thing in common—inflammation.

So if we can treat inflammation, we can do away with these ailments. Simple, right?

But here's the thing: glucosamine and chondroitin—the most common natural products used to treat joint deterioration and pain do not have the power to correct inflammation in the joints.

Joint remedies that actually do the job need to address the cause of joint damage. And the fact is that inflammation plays a central role.

Here's what you need to know about joints and bones, and why you can't treat joint pain effectively without treating inflammation:

1. Our body is constantly absorbing and replacing old bone with new, healthy bone.

2. Where one bone meets another, the bones are covered in cushioning called cartilage. This keeps bones from rubbing against each other.

3. Cartilage is nourished by fluid called synovial fluid, which fills the spaces in the joints, between the bones.

4. When the joints are inflamed, cartilage can't get the nourishment it needs from the synovial fluid. So inflammation destroys normal cartilage tissue and gets in the way of new, healthy cartilage being formed.

5. If inflammation is controlled, the body can again begin forming and nourishing new, healthy cartilage. The result? Normal, healthy, comfortable joints.

In some cases of joint pain, such as rheumatoid arthritis, inflammation comes first and destroys cartilage and—if left unchecked—bone.

In other cases, like osteoarthritis, the "wear and tear" destruction of cartilage leads to inflammation in the joint tissues. Either way, what results is a vicious cycle that can only be interrupted in one way: by controlling inflammation.

Here's why that's so important: once you control inflammation, the damaged joints and underlying bones can begin to heal themselves. This self-healing ability of bones and joints is the basis of all natural healing in all tissues of the body. No matter how many so-called bone-supporting nutrients you pour into the system (assuming they even make it into your joints), they won't work if you don't stop the inflammation cycle.

Can your body even use glucosamine and chondroitin?

Many doctors and medical scientists have questioned for decades whether glucosamine (a sugar amine) is even sufficiently absorbed into the joint tissues, believing that it is destroyed in the gastrointestinal tract and/or the bloodstream before it can even enter the joints. It is, after all, a combination of glucose or sugar (which is readily metabolized for energy) and an amine, which like most protein constituents, are broken apart by digestion and enzymes.

Chondroitin comes with its own list of issues. Concerns have been raised about the source it comes from and how well the body can actually absorb it, and to what extent. It seems like most all the "new" discoveries over the years when it comes to chondroitin have to do with some new, exotic species or location from which this common natural substance is harvested. This has made for some putatively attractive marketing pitches...but not evidence that it is absorbed into the body and actually works for joint pain. That's why chondroitin has become widely regarded in the medical community as worthless.

Side effects of glucosamine include digestive complaints such as abdominal pain, poor appetite, nausea, heartburn, constipation, diarrhea, and vomiting. Which makes sense for something that is not being absorbed properly in the gastrointestinal tract.

History holds the secret to joint relief

Modern science is proving what our ancestors knew: Natural remedies can curb inflammation and promote bone and joint health.

Do you remember what the wise men brought as gifts to celebrate the birth of Jesus? Gold, frankincense, and myrrh. Believe it or not, all three of those are proven arthritis remedies (and you can trust men who just walked halfway around the world to know what soothes achy joints!). No wonder they were so valuable.

Gold injected into the joints actually does help arthritis, but its expense puts it out of reach for most of us. Frankincense and myrrh, on the other hand, have a long history in supporting joints—and new research continues to support their use.

Frankincense, also known as **Boswellia**, is best known in the West as a potent incense that fills churches with a familiar fragrance. But far beyond smelling good, frankincense is valued for its medicinal properties. In fact, it has held an important place in Asian medicine for millennia. Ayurvedic practitioners have known for ages that Boswellia is a key treatment for joints. And the reason it works: It stops inflammation.

And, again, that allows your cartilage to rebuild itself. Like most natural healing, rebuilding healthy bone and cartilage to a permanent solution is a slow and steady process that takes time. But if you take care of the inflammation in the meantime, it helps stop the pain and increases mobility, while allowing the joint to repair itself over time.

Myrrh, found in abundance in the Middle East, is valued for its anti- inflammatory effects too. In fact, it's held in such high esteem that it was one of the gifts the Queen of Sheba brought to King Solomon.

Vitamin C (500 mg/day), *vitamin D* (2,000 IU/day), and *vitamin E* (400 to 600 IU/day—see page 106 for further explanation on dosage information) are always important for bone and joint health. And yes, you need all three to work best together.

Capsicum frutescens **(cayenne pepper)**. You generally see capsaicin as an ingredient in topical creams (usually in 0.025% and 0.075% strengths). They can be very effective for relieving joint pain. However eating red chili peppers (if you like spicy food) can also have remarkably beneficial effects.

Curcuma longa **(turmeric)** The active ingredient, curcumin, of this commonly used spice has anti-inflammatory and lipid-lowering effects. It is one of the three common components of traditional curry spice (together with coriander and cumin, and sometimes red chili pepper). Curcumin's lipid-lowering effects observed in animal experiments are attributed to changes in fatty acid metabolism and facilitating the conversion of cholesterol to bile acids. There are also reports of its benefit in patients with osteoarthritis. The benefit of turmeric is not conclusively proven but its use as a spice in an overall healthy diet is appropriate. Curcumin supplements are widely available in natural food stores and online supplement retailers. A good general dose is 200 mg per day.

Withania somnifera **(winter cherry)**. Basic science studies suggest that this herb may have anti-inflammatory, antioxidant, immune-modulatory and anti-aging properties. It might also have a positive influence on the endocrine and central nervous systems. The mechanisms of these proposed actions require additional clarification. Several observational and randomized studies have reported its usefulness in the treatment of arthritic conditions

Zingiber officinale **(ginger)**. Ginger is widely used in Asia, most commonly for control of nausea and osteoarthritis pain. Several randomized trials have shown its benefit in controlling nausea associated with pregnancy, motion sickness and anesthesia, and some studies have demonstrated its usefulness in the treatment of osteoarthritis.

Omega-3 fatty acids. The essential fatty acids in fish oil are another tremendous natural anti-inflammatory. However, to get as much as you need—3 to 10 grams per day—you'll likely need to increase the amount of omega-3 containing foods you eat (like salmon, sardines, and walnuts) and take a fish oil supplement as well. Fish oil supplements are widely available. Just be sure to look for one that contains both the DHA and EPA fatty acids.

It should be mentioned that the methodology and quality of many studies aimed at determining the effectiveness of various herbs are less than satisfactory. Also, many studies involve the use of preparations which contain several herbs and other nutrients, which is quite common in herbal practice. While such trials are useful, they do not, in and of themselves, identify and discern the beneficial effects of specific herbs. In one such trial involving a combination preparation of Withiania somnifera, Bosweillia serrata, Curcuma longa, and zinc, osteoarthritis patients reported a significant reduction in their level of pain compared to those in the control group.

If you're looking for a joint supplement, you'd do well to find one that has these potent herbal anti-inflammatories, as well as some specific nutrients whose effectiveness is proven by modern science.

Chapter 14

Rheumatoid arthritis: One of medicine's most agonizing mysteries—UNRAVELED!

Modern medicine botches a lot of things. But the way it treats rheumatoid arthritis may be one of the worst examples.

For centuries, rheumatoid arthritis (RA) has largely been a mystery. A very painful one at that.

The problem is, once again, that western medicine only focuses on ONE aspect of the disease.

Modern medicine has classified RA as an auto-immune disease. Of course, when I was in training during the 1970s, that's what the experts ended up calling a lot of diseases they simply didn't understand.

Today, we know there is indeed an immune component involved in rheumatoid arthritis (RA). But, as is the case in many other auto-immune disorders, there's also a strong mind- body connection. And, more recently, yet another factor has come to light—the nervous system connection.

Finding real relief from this mysterious chronic condition requires treating all three aspects. Unfortunately, most doctors simply aren't.

That said, make no mistake: RA is a dangerous systemic condition that requires management by a competent rheumatologist. And the good news is, more and more doctors are recognizing that there are also complementary approaches that can help soothe RA. More on that in just a minute. First, it's important to understand how it all ties together.

It's all connected

I talk a lot about the mind- body connection in my *Insiders' Cures* newsletter. But I have to—because western science separated the two long ago. And that was—and is—a huge mistake. Other ethno-medical traditions in Asia and around the world never separated them. This is one reason these other medical traditions appear more "wholistic" to us today.

But even based on modern science, growing evidence shows the mind and body are linked—or "married." For better or worse, in sickness and in health.

It boils down to three inter- connected components:

1 "Psycho"—the mind/brain connection

2. "Neuro"—the nervous system connection

3. "Immunology"—the immune system connection

In fact, today there's an entire field of medicine called "psycho-neuro-immunology." Which provides a tangible scientific approach, a physiologic model, and a growing body of data proving the mind-body connections.

Here's how each component works…

For the "psycho" component, we know that the mind-brain is connected through thoughts, emotional feelings, and levels of consciousness to influence the body. But it's not just a one-way street. The biochemicals, called neuro-peptides, that we associate as being in the brain, such as neurotransmitters, are actually present throughout the body. In fact, neurotransmitters are found in even greater quantities in the gut, for example, than they are in the nervous system.

Further, the production of specific hormones (which occurs throughout the body in the thyroid, pancreas, adrenal glands, and ovaries or testes) is controlled by specific neuro- peptides released by the pituitary gland of the brain. These hormones are released into the circulatory system and carried to all parts of the body in the blood.

For the "neuro" part of the equation, the nervous system originates in the brain and spinal cord as well. Nerves also travel to all parts of the body, both sensing and influencing all tissues at both voluntary (conscious) and involuntary (unconscious) levels.

But now there's a third piece being added to the puzzle— "immunology."

Like neuro-peptides and nerves, the immune system is also present throughout the body. Immune cells (white blood cells) travel throughout the blood. And there are specialized concentrations of these cells in the adenoids, tonsils, spleen, appendix, and throughout the gastrointestinal tract (without fully understanding their role, 20th century surgeons considered them all to be expendable). They are also concentrated in the thymus gland during childhood.

When you look at how each of these three components impacts the body from head-to-toe on their own…it's not hard to see how they are all inter-related as well. The psycho-neuro-immunology-connection becomes quite apparent.

So what causes rheumatoid arthritis?

One way the immune system works is by making antibodies that match to antigens on invading bacteria and viruses. Antigens are foreign substances that stimulate the immune system. The antibodies attack the antigens and then white blood cells can destroy the microbes.

These microbial antigens are often made up of proteins and/ or polysaccharides that are commonly found in nature. These are some of the same proteins and polysaccharides that exist in normal, healthy biological substances as well. Unfortunately, when the immune system can get out of synch, some of the antibodies it makes against microbes get confused and cross-react with certain normal tissues. Thus, the immune system can attack our own bodies—causing an "auto" immune disease.

RA is the result of your immune system attacking the cartilage in your joints. This confusion can stem from a true bacterial infection, like "rheumatic fever." Or it can appear more mysteriously from a stress-related immune imbalance—this is the mind-body-immune connection.

While there is accordingly a mind-body component, caution must be exercised with rheumatoid arthritis. It causes real, physical damage with serious complications that require experienced medical management. The best thing you can do is to consult a rheumatologist who can help determine which of the drugs for RA appear to be safe, effective, and appropriate for you. And whether there older ones that are more reliable (as in the case with blood pressure medications).

That said, doctors and patients alike are realizing that there are also natural approaches you can take to help alleviate RA. Especially when it comes to addressing the mind- body connection.

True "complements" to RA treatment

A wide range of "mind-body" approaches can reduce the stress that inevitably accompanies the pain with which RA patients struggle on a daily basis. For those best suited to your emotional type take the short quiz featured on www.drmicozzi.com, or in my book with Michael Jawer *Your Emotional Type*.

Gentle movements—as in traditional yoga or tai chi—can also be helpful. Likewise, swimming can provide just the right kind of low-stress movement and physical exercise. Light massage, low-impact exercise, and just getting outdoors (walking, riding a bike, or light gardening) can also be good.

For the pain itself, acupuncture can often work wonders.

In China and India, rheumatic conditions are associated with "cold and damp." So while the inflammation may seem hot, it actually helps to seek warmth and avoid cold and damp circumstances and climates. In fact, one ancient Ayurvedic treatment involves immersing the joints in warm sand.

This can easily be accomplished on a sunny beach (while also providing you, and your bones and joints, with some much-needed vitamin D).

Whatever complementary therapy you decide to try, don't go it alone. The best way to ensure you get the most relief is to work with a rheumatologist who can recommend the best complementary therapies for your particular needs.

Chapter 15

What you need to know about NSAIDs

Obviously, for mainstream medicine, figuring out how to effectively treat pain can be a real...pain.

This is especially true when doctors persist in ignoring all of the natural approaches for pain management, and slavishly comply with all of the political prohibitions placed on effective pain relievers by big government regulators and armed law enforcement. Suddenly, these doctors find they don't have many good options left. So it's no surprise that their desperate patients turn to over-the-counter pain remedies. But there are some important things you need to know about these pain relievers.

The common painkiller you should avoid at all costs

Fortunately, there are some over-the-counter drug and herbal remedies that are effective—and *safe*—anti-inflammatory agents. But you may be surprised to learn that Tylenol (acetaminophen) is not among them.

Also known as paracetamol, acetaminophen was originally an industrial chemical developed in Germany. Since then, it has caused more pain than it has cured. In fact, it has become the leading cause of acute liver failure in the United States.

Tylenol was actually one of the first drugs for which we developed protocols to monitor therapeutic and toxic blood levels when I worked with a technical team at McDonnell Douglas (now Boeing) on instrumentation from the manned space program.

Our job was to adapt analytical technology from the NASA space exploration program to everyday clinical use. We were also looking at other potent and potentially dangerous drugs, like anticonvulsants, amphetamines, barbiturates and psychoactive drugs. That's right: All of these dangerous toxic potential killers were treated in the same category as a common household pain-reliever.

I have known otherwise intelligent people who kept taking more and more Tylenol until their knee pain went away…just so they could keep their appointments to play handball or basketball. They may have won the match, but at what cost? I guarantee you they won't be thinking about those victories when they're diagnosed with liver failure.

Acetaminophen found worthless for pain besides being highly toxic

Well, now doctors have come out with a second opinion about acetaminophen (Tylenol). For years, everyone has admitted it is the leading cause of liver toxicity and fatal liver failure in the US today. Now they have a second opinion; it's also <u>worthless</u> for pain!

An important new study found the use of acetaminophen for the most common cause of pain and disability in working Americans was no more effective than placebo, or taking a sugar pill.[5] The drug was worthless whether it was taken regularly three times every day (3,990 mg total, or nearly 4 grams—more like a food quantity than a drug), or only taken when needed.

Patients taking this drug, whether on the 4 gram per day regular schedule or only as needed, suffered an average of 17 days before recovering from a bout of disabling back pain.

But patients taking a sugar pill took only 16 days to recover!

The drug actually made patients spend an extra day in pain and disabled, missing work, or school, or daily activities. To someone suffering from back pain spending that 17th day in pain by taking Tylenol can seem like an eternity.

So, that's what you get for your trouble and expense, not to mention risking liver failure. You get to spend <u>an extra day</u> in pain before recovering.

Since Tylenol is a metabolic poison, I suspect it actually interferes with your body's normal ability to heal naturally and safely—and delays your healing by one day while doing nothing to help you.

This group of researchers from Australia had previously conducted an analysis of prior studies that found no benefits to the use of this drug. To further their analysis of this gap, they enlisted 1,643 participants of average age 45 years from 235 pain centers in Australia in the Paracetamol for Low Back Pain (PACE) trial. Note:

Acetaminophen is known as Paracetamol outside the US (like a criminal fugitive, it goes by aliases, perhaps for the same reason).

There were no benefits to the drug in any of the studies. The researchers did provide good quality advice and reassurance to all study participants, a feature that is often absent from usual care.

The scandal is that universal medical practice guidelines for management of low back pain call for the first-line use of this toxic drug. You have to wonder where that idea came from?

The researchers point out, that despite the "universal" acceptance for the first use of Tylenol , there was <u>never</u> any good evidence for it—leading to their review analysis and then to their clinical trial.

So, what was all that about the importance of so-called "evidence-based" medical practice? What a painful scandal.

The mainstream management of low back pain was never any good—at least when left in the hands of drugs or surgeries.

And acetaminophen was never a good drug based on its toxicity alone. The new evidence that it doesn't even work; makes this drug a big "less-than-zero" as far its therapeutic index of benefits versus risks.

A safer way to find OTC pain relief

While I urge you never to take Tylenol, I have found ibuprofen drugs like Advil and Motrin to be effective pain relievers when nothing else works.

The key is to be vigilant against these drugs' alarming side effects, and to carefully monitor your dosages.

Ibuprofen, along with aspirin, naproxen (Aleve), and a whole host of prescription drugs, is part of a class of pain relievers known as NSAIDs (non-steroidal anti-inflammatory drugs). Many of these drugs came onto the scene during the 1980s and were quickly accepted by people seeking pain relief.

However, NSAIDS are associated with dangerous side effects in the gastrointestinal tract, including ulcers, bleeding, and colon perforations. These drugs can wreak havoc all the way through the average 26-foot length of the GI tract. That's a lot of territory for damage to occur.

Alarmingly, these problems are not rare. In fact, about 1 to 2 percent of routine NSAID users experience GI complications that are so severe, they have to be hospitalized.[6] And if you're older than 65, have a history of peptic ulcers, take NSAIDS and anticoagulants at the same time, or pop an NSAID when you're taking a daily aspirin, you may be particularly susceptible to these complications.

The good news is, at recommended doses, ibuprofen is the least likely of the NSAIDs to cause these side effects. But while you don't want to take too much of this painkiller, you also don't want to take too little.

Ibuprofen is still available as a prescription pain reliever, and an effective dose is considered to be one or two 800 mg tablets. Compare that to the puny 200 mg in the Advil or Motrin tablets you buy at the drug store. I've found that when ibuprofen does not provide fast, effective pain relief, it's often because the doses in these over-the-counter products are simply too low.

Of course, I always recommend trying natural pain relievers first. But if you choose to use NSAIDs, make sure to let your doctor know. You should also keep an eye out for signs of GI bleeding, including dark stools or blood in your toilet.

BRAIN-HEALERS FROM BEHIND THE CURTAIN

Part 3: Brain-healers from behind the curtain

Chapter 16
The Insider's Answer for Dodging Dementia

Brain deficiencies and disorders have been a mystery to medicine for centuries. In fact, scientists are just as puzzled about "mental health" and disease today as they were a hundred years ago. This is despite the efforts of our recent politically-designated "Decade of the Brain" (1990-1999). Unfortunately we've yet to overcome this century-long challenge despite the lavish funds poured into the usual academic-medical complex.

Years ago, many mental illnesses were thought to have an underlying disease (or pathology). If an underlying disease could be found, then a treatment could be developed. Sigmund Freud originally became a brain pathologist, searching for these organic causes. But when the brains of people with mental illnesses were found to be "normal" pathologically, he eventually switched courses. This is how he came to establish psychoanalysis as a different path to understanding mental health.

On the other side of the equation, brain disorders that, in fact, turned out to have an underlying pathological cause were mistakenly thought to be psychological illnesses. For example, "general paresis of the insane" turned out to be caused by tertiary syphilis, where the untreated syphilis organisms go on to destroy brain tissue.

Modern psychiatry still struggles with how to diagnose and classify brain disorders. Periodically they issue a new edition of the *Diagnostic and Statistical Manual* (DSM), the "bible of mental health." But lacking an understanding of the mechanisms of many disorders, we fall back on using statistical descriptions and characteristics.

In addition, the process for updating the DSM for 2012 has been fraught with conflict and dissension, as documented in the popular press. And of course, it's all due to the same problems we find throughout modern medical research: academic careerism, medicalization of life events and processes (which particularly have an impact on how people are "feeling"), limitations in research methodology, government interference with professional practices, politicization and political correctness, and the bias to replace psychotherapies with psychiatric drug therapies.

Another part of the problem is the large and powerful organization of professional psychologists. While they do not use psychiatric drugs, they have been slow to embrace the kind of "mind-body" therapies that have been effective for problems that seem to cross the border between mind, body, and spirit (although they politely gave audiences to me and my colleagues, and our medical textbooks, at their annual meetings through the 2000's).

And of course all the while, research, development, and discovery of effective treatments for you slog on at a snail's pace.

So what, exactly, DO we know?

All confusion and debate aside, thankfully, there are some important fundamentals about how the brain works that are central to understanding the similarities and differences inherent in brain biology.

The brain is very metabolically active. Therefore, it needs a constant supply of a lot of blood to deliver oxygen and glucose to support brain metabolism. One-third of total blood volume flows to the brain. That means one-third of the blood cells, one-third of the oxygen, one-third of the blood sugar and other nutrients circulating in our blood is needed by the brain.

Accordingly, the brain is very sensitive to deprivation of oxygen, glucose, and nutrients. In fact, the brain will die if deprived of oxygen and glucose for only 2-3 minutes (loss of consciousness, coma, then death). This is a striking difference when compared to the needs of the lower body. For example, during surgery, when blood flow is clamped off below the kidneys, the legs can go without oxygen for hours and return to normal health as long as blood flow is eventually restored.

The brain is also very selective in what it allows to pass from the blood into the brain tissue. This is something we refer to as the "blood-brain barrier." While other tissues of the body are generally bathed in the same constituents that are carried in the blood, the brain carefully selects what is allowed to pass into the fluids that surround the brain (cerebro-spinal fluid). This property is fortunate because it keeps out a lot of toxins that would be harmful to the sensitive brain tissue.

This selective nature of the brain becomes critical when it comes to medications that are prescribed for mental health and disease. At the same time, it's important to make sure any nutrients you may be taking are in forms that will make it across the highly selective blood-brain barrier.

Neuro-nutritive nutrients for your body and mind

There are many approaches to maintaining health and managing diseases of the body using herbal and dietary supplements. However, when it comes to understanding and applying basic nutrition to enhancing and improving the normal mental functions and performance of the mind, there is still the "blood-brain barrier" to contend with. The good news is, it *can* be done.

Through the combination of cognitive science and nutritional medicine, science has developed dietary supplements and food products that can enhance basic brain and mental function and performance. While there is much *talk* of "smart drugs," which may theoretically be taken by anyone to support improved mental performance, there is some *proof* of smart nutrients that cross the blood-brain barrier and help the brain do its basic job using safe and effective vitamins, minerals, and natural constituents.

Unfortunately, many of these natural "smart nutrients" are still clouded in controversy. Fielding heavy criticism from the modern medical-complex. So much so, that many "alternative" practitioners will even avoid the topic completely.

Even herbs that have been used effectively for decades—such as *ginkgo biloba* for dementia, *kava kava* for anxiety, *St John's wort* for mild-moderate depression, *valerian* for insomnia, and *feverfew* for migraine headache. So you can imagine that when it comes to addressing something as serious, and confounding, as Alzheimer's disease, nearly everyone looks the other way. Which is tragic because currently, it's estimated that nearly 5 million Americans have Alzheimer's Disease (AD). It's also the 8th leading cause of death in the United States. And once diagnosed, the average life span of an Alzheimer's patient is eight years. The spectrum (and fearful specter) of age-related cognitive decline is a major neuropsychological area that has yet to be addressed by the pharmaceutical or the natural products industry.

But there are alternatives that may help.

And recently, the research behind one nutrient in particular is beginning to lead the pack...see the next chapter for details.

Three more common causes of dementia

Alzheimer's is just one *form* of devastating dementia. There are three other common neuro-degenerative problems afflicting the brain and mind. The common denominator in all dementia is neuro-degeneration, destruction and loss of neurons, or nerve cells in the brain.

Schizophrenia-related cognitive impairment. Today as many as 60 million people worldwide have schizophrenia. Most people with schizophrenia also suffer from cognitive impairment, although it is independent of the psychotic symptoms of the illness. In North America, it is estimated that more than two million people have schizophrenia. While there is an $18-billion drug business to treat the psychosis associated with schizophrenia, there are no approved drugs for treating the cognitive impairment.

Mild cognitive impairment from bypass surgery. Approximately 500,000 patients in the U.S. and 800,000 patients worldwide undergo coronary artery bypass graft (CABG) surgery every year. It has now been recognized that the changes in blood flow associated with the procedure bring about dementia in many patients. Currently there is no therapy available approved to ameliorate or treat the cognitive damage associated with artery bypass surgery.

Stroke. Every 45 seconds in the U.S., someone experiences a stroke. This fact translates into approximately 700,000 new or recurrent strokes in the U.S. each year. It is the second leading cause of mortality in the world, the third leading cause of death in the U.S., and is the leading cause of long-term disability. In spite of this, there has been failure to provide effective treatments.

Type III diabetes–the brand new, DEADLY epidemic no one saw coming

You've probably heard the old saying "bad things come in threes." And after nearly a century of research, it appears that may be the case with diabetes.

You're likely familiar with Type I and Type II diabetes. But now it looks like there's yet another form on the horizon—Type III diabetes. And it may be the most sinister, dangerous form of the disease yet.

A modern-day disaster 90 years in the making

For centuries diabetes had been known primarily as a condition of excess fluid loss through frequent urination, with sugar in the urine.

But in 1922, two researchers won a Nobel prize when they discovered that diabetes mellitus was a primary deficiency of insulin. Insulin is responsible for moving glucose (sugar) from the blood into the tissues. Without it, the tissues, including the brain, literally starve to death in a sea of plenty.

Since then, there have been many more discoveries regarding this condition. Like the difference between Type I and Type II diabetes.

The Nobel-prize winning researchers discovered what has come to be known as Type I (or "juvenile") diabetes. With Type I, from childhood, the pancreas simply does not make insulin. Type I diabetes is treatable by injecting synthetic insulin over regular time intervals.

But as the 20th century progressed, an initially mysterious new type of diabetes emerged. People with this form of the disease produce adequate insulin. But their tissues become resistant to the actions of that insulin. And, as a result, glucose can't enter the tissues. Instead, it accumulates in the blood. This "insulin-resistant" diabetes became known as Type II diabetes.

Now, I believe we are witnessing a third form of the disease—Type III diabetes. And it may have been masquerading as the No. 1 medical mystery of our time—the modern misery of Alzheimer's Disease.

Elevated blood sugar shrinks your brain A recent Australian study found that high blood sugar levels appear to actually cause the brain to shrink.[1]

Even in people who don't have Type I or Type II diabetes.

This study of 250 men and women showed that high blood sugar levels appear to damage the brain. Specifically, they cause the areas associated with memory, cognitive function, and emotional processing to shrink. And impairments in these areas are the hallmark symptoms of Alzheimer's dementia.

In fact, these researchers found that highly-educated people in their 60s, with even mildly elevated blood sugar, had the brains of unhealthy people in their 70s.

While prior studies have shown that diabetics have higher rates of dementia, this is the first study to show these effects <u>even in people who are not diagnosed as having Type I or Type II diabetes</u>. So, are they suffering from Type III diabetes?

In non-Type I or -Type II diabetics, high blood sugar can result not only from consuming too much sugar in the diet, but from generally poor diet, lack of exercise, and chronic stress. So, blood sugar is a problem for *everyone*, not just diabetics. And now we're seeing just how significantly it can affect your brain (as well as other parts of your body).

I first heard about this link last September, and have been looking into it ever since. And, indeed, a large body of evidence is now suggesting that Alzheimer's is primarily a metabolic disease, just like diabetes. But different enough from the already well-known Types I and II to warrant its own classification. Type III diabetes.

Why your brain needs insulin

As I mentioned above, an association between Alzheimer's dementia and Type II diabetes is already long-established. In fact, the risk of dementia among Type II diabetics is *two to three times higher* than in the general population. There are also associations between Alzheimer's and obesity, and Alzheimer's and metabolic syndrome (a pattern of diet- and metabolic- related disorders).

Some researchers first proposed that Alzheimer's was actually another form of diabetes back in 2005.[2] The authors of these original studies investigated the brains of people who had died of dementia. They found that the levels of both insulin and insulin-like growth factors in the brains of Alzheimer's patients were sharply reduced. And insulin levels were lowest in the parts of the brain that appeared most affected by dementia.

Insulin in the brain has a number of important functions in addition to glucose metabolism. It helps regulate transmission of signals from one neuron (nerve cell) to another. And it influences their growth as well as their ability to adapt to changes and survive.

Experiments conducted since then appear to support the link between diet and dementia. As ever, these observations show the biochemistry of dementia to be fantastically complex, involving inflammation, stress, oxidation, the accumulation of a certain brain protein and the transformation of another—among other factors. This is one case where more research does, in fact, need to be done. And this is the kind of research that NIH should really be doing.

However, if current indications hold true, Alzheimer's disease could be yet another catastrophic impact of poor diets.

Perhaps one of the worst thus far Around 35 million people suffer from Alzheimer's disease worldwide and based on current projections, with the rate at which the population is aging, this epidemic will rise to 100 million by 2050.

But if, as many scientists now believe, it is caused largely by the brain's impaired response to insulin, those numbers could rise much further. In the U.S., the percentage of the population with Type II diabetes has almost tripled in just 30 years.

If Alzheimer's dementia—Type III diabetes—acts the same way, the potential for more human suffering is immense.

But while U.S. government research on Alzheimer's flounders around, there are steps you can take to help protect yourself and your family now. In fact, there are some exceptionally effective tools for combating this burgeoning epidemic.

Starting with one that I'm particularly excited about.

The latest blood-sugar darling tackles Alzheimer's, too

Berberine is quickly becoming one of the new "darlings" of the nutritional medicine world. And the "buzz" has focused largely on this herbal remedy's ability to balance blood sugar and combat diabetes. But the new research on berberine that caught my eye recently had nothing to do with blood sugar or diabetes—or so I initially thought.

Several new studies have shown impressive results using berberine for Alzheimer's. [3,4,5]

But now that Alzheimer's is emerging as Type III diabetes, the link between these two fields of research on berberine makes perfect sense.

But berberine defends against Alzheimer's not only by helping to regulate blood sugar.

3-tiered brain protection you won't find anywhere else

New experimental results have found that berberine protects the brain in at least three more distinct ways:

1. It can safeguard your brain from the dangerous oxidation damage

that can "eat away" at brain tissue.

2. It targets and destroys memory- killing enzymes that have long been considered key in the development of Alzheimer's.

3. It promotes healthy blood flow directly to the brain—an essential element to conquering dementia.

Berberine also seems to be able to block certain nerve receptors, which may partly explain its anti-Alzheimer and neurotransmitter-modulating properties.

Add these specific actions to berberine's well-established blood sugar benefits and it appears that this herb may hold the key to preventing and even slowing the progression of Alzheimer's disease (Type III diabetes) like nothing before it.

I recommend 500 mg per day, taken over the course of two or three doses to achieve a steady state.

The first step in avoiding and managing ANY type of diabetes

Of course, no discussion of metabolic disorders is complete without addressing the importance of diet.

The food industry engineers its products to bypass the neurological signals that would otherwise prompt people to stop eating. Filling them with unhealthy fats, sugars, and high fructose corn syrup. Essentially ensuring they're completely devoid of any real nutrients. Which makes processed, packaged foods a disaster not just for your waistline, but also for your blood sugar, your brain—and your health in general.

Cutting out overly processed foods should be the first step in avoiding— or treating—ANY disease, including diabetes (Types I, II, and III).

Chapter 17

Berberine—the Alzheimer's answer no one will pay attention to

Berberine is a mental powerhouse that may have the ability on almost all fronts to provide greater cognitive support and protection. To dodge dementia before it stops you. And it's a solution you aren't likely to hear about elsewhere.

Berberine has long been used throughout history. It is still used today in Northern India, as a bright yellow coloring dye for leather, wood, and wool fabrics. In fact, if you have a woven Indian carpet on your floor, you have probably already noted the bright yellow color imparted by berberine. It also has a use in modern medicine and pathology because of its ability to stain certain tissue cells to show their appearance under the microscope.

Berberine is found in numerous plants worldwide, including the large plant family *Berberis*, or the barberries. It is also found in the important (and ecologically threatened) medicinal plant *Hydrastis canadensis* (Goldenseal), and the important Chinese herb *Rhizome coptidis* (Golden thread or *Huang-Lian*), among others. Berberine is usually found in the roots, stems, and bark. Chemically, it is an isoquinolone alkaloid, and the plant alkaloids are known to have a number of potent biological activities.

Indeed, typical of plant alkaloids, berberine has a number of health effects, throughout the body, including acting as a potent antibiotic (which can also overcome infections caused by bacteria that are resistant to drug antibiotics), anti-fungal, and anti-parasitic.

Hundreds of recent research studies (far too many to share in detail here) reveals this medical marvel can provide a host of additional health benefits. It's been shown to help lower cholesterol, improve blood sugar metabolism, and has anti-cancer properties.

And incredibly, new research shows berberine may also hold the key to preventing and even slowing the progression of Alzheimer's disease and other dementia, like nothing before it. In part, because berberine has been found to be able to penetrate the blood-brain barrier and effect cells of the central nervous system. And new experimental results have found that berberine works in three distinct ways:

1. It can safeguard your brain from the dangerous oxidation damage that can "eat away" at brain tissue.

2. It targets and destroys memory-killing enzymes that have long thought to be key in the development of Alzheimer's.

3. It promotes healthy blood flow directly to the brain—an essential element to conquering dementia.

Berberine also seems to be able to block certain nerve receptors, which may partly explain its anti-Alzheimer's and neurotransmitter modulating properties. Other experimental studies have shown berberine to increase neurotransmitter (noradrenaline and serotonin) levels in the brain. Berberine may also act in a manner comparable to some anti-depressant drugs by increasing available serotonin in the brain.

Results suggest benefits in patients with depression, bipolar affective disorder, schizophrenia, or related diseases in which cognitive capabilities are affected.

The half-life of berberine suggests administration of a daily dose of 500 mg, taken two or three times per day to achieve a steady state.

7 simple tips for spotting early signs of Alzheimer's disease

As I've mentioned before, recent research indicates you are the best expert there is when it comes to early detection of Alzheimer's disease (AD).

And that's great news. Because early detection is crucial with

AD. And the sooner you spot the problem, the sooner you can do something about it. In fact, keep reading and I'll tell you more about a natural powerhouse that can help prevent and slow the progression of Alzheimer's disease.

But first, take this short quiz. It will help you assess the difference between normal, age-related memory loss and cognitive decline due to Alzheimer's disease.

1. Are all new signs of memory lapses significant for dementia?

Answer: No.

It's very typical to forget names, dates, and appointments as you get older. These "signs" may be part of a lifelong pattern. These changes have more to do with neural organization than degeneration. But if you have to ask for the <u>same</u> information, over and over, that is not typical. Also, take note if you need to rely more heavily on memory aids. Or, do you frequently forget regular dates, like the day of the week the trash truck comes?

2. If I misplace objects more often, is that an early sign of dementia?

Answer: It depends.

Misplacing objects frequently is more likely due to distraction rather than dementia. But if you frequently have to <u>replace</u> missing eyeglasses, checkbooks, keys, jackets, etc. it's time to get a formal cognitive assessment. In addition, if you find lost objects in strange places, that can also signal cognitive decline. For example, if you find your car keys in the bathroom cabinet or in the dishwasher.

3. Which speech pattern is a sign of dementia?

    a. speaking clearly and concisely

    b. rambling on, frequently forgetting words or phrases

    c. not recalling a word or two

    d. all of the above

Answer: B.

Forgetting a word or searching for the right word is a typical part of everyday life. But consistently struggling with the same word or words repeatedly is a sign of cognitive decline.

4. **Which is a sign of cognitive decline?**

    a. Taking a wrong turn in a familiar area

    b. Getting lost driving in a new area using a map

    c. Never having any idea where you are unless using a GPS device to tell you

    d. Frequently getting lost in familiar areas

Answer: D.

Getting lost in familiar places while walking or driving is a strong sign of cognitive decline. But remember to check on the many cognitive side effects from drugs, which may be responsible and are reversible. This problem happens especially among older adults who take multiple drugs.

5. **I habitually miss bill payments and appointments. Does this mean I might have Alzheimer's disease?**

    Answer: Again, it depends.

Missing appointments and bill payments can happen to anyone at any age. But an increased pattern can signal a decline in cognitive function. However, these lapses can also happen with mood dysfunction. So, take this question to a deeper level…does it take you much longer to pay the bills or work on your budget? Or do you now have trouble adding a group of numbers accurately? These changes may indicate a problem with cognition.

6. **It takes me longer to complete routine tasks. Isn't this just normal aging?**

    Answer: Maybe not.

Studies show that when you multitask, you actually work more slowly. So don't try to balance your checkbook while watching TV and talking on the phone. It will take you longer. If you want to finish more quickly, focus your efforts on one activity at a time. If you still have trouble performing a single routine task like following a favorite recipe, it may signal more significant memory problems.

7. **I react to everyday stresses with greater anxiety, anger, depression, and/or mood swings than ever before. Is this a normal part of aging?**

Answer: No.

Typically, we learn to handle emotions better as we age. But some people never learn. And in some, exaggerated emotional responses may indicate the onset of progressive cognitive decline. People with Alzheimer's disease rely on routines to go about their day. They may become irritable or uncomfortable when their routine changes for any reason. As a result, they may begin to withdraw from social experiences they once enjoyed.

If any of the scenarios above sound familiar, don't ignore them! Talk about your concerns with friends and family.

And the sooner you act, the better!

Chapter 18

Beyond berberine: Your nutrient toolbox for cognitive support

As mentioned above, there are several natural products that have been shown to help protect the brain. Following is a quick list of those least talked about in terms of brain function and mental health by both mainstream and alternative practitioners.

Creatine

Creatine is a beta-amino acid popularized in recent years by bodybuilders and other athletes for muscle development and repair of muscle tissue after exercise, as well as energy-enhancing properties. Some reports suggest that people over 60 do not make enough creatine to maintain muscle and strength.

But creatine is becoming more widely researched for its neuro-protective and neurogenesis benefits. For example, as an element for some alternative treatments for Amyotrophic Lateral Sclerosis (ALS) and Parkinson's disease. The dosages for such treatment would be at a higher, therapeutic level, and not the more typical recommended dose of between 1 and 2 grams. Accordingly, use of creatine should be individually tailored and monitored under supervision of a qualified health practitioner.

Lecithin

Lecithin is generally a mixture of glycolipids, triglycerides, and phospholipids (e.g. phosphatidylcholine, phosphatidylethanolamine, and phosphatidylinositol). Phospholipids are the major component of the membranes that encase every cell in the body. In the brain, phosphatidylcholine and phosphatidylinositol protect nerve cells by forming a protective sheath around them to insulate them, allowing nerve impulses to move more efficiently to and between cells. In addition, phosphatidylcholine is a precursor of acetylcholine, a neurotransmitter in the brain and muscles. An increase in acetylcholine may lead to more efficient nerve and muscle function and increased memory performance and capacity. Unfortunately, some medications can deplete acetylcholine. Supplementing with lecithin may help counter this drug side effect.

Some qualitative research on lecithin supplementation found that when a short-term or long-term memory deficit exists, a single therapeutic dose of lecithin can increase memory performance within 90 minutes. It may also help improve verbal and visual memory. And has neuro-protective effects related to Alzheimer's disease.

Lecithin is available in 1,000 mg supplement doses, but may require up to 25 grams (25,000 mg) daily, used in food quantities, to see the full benefits.

Royal Jelly

Royal jelly is an amino acid-rich gelatinous substance secreted by worker bees to feed queen bees. Since queen bees grow to be considerably larger than worker bees, and live much longer, it has been assumed by many enthusiasts to produce benefits for humans. The popularity of health products containing royal jelly has increased over the past years. While its anti-aging and energy-enhancing properties have been reputed for many decades, only recently has more rigorous research been performed to separate fact from folklore.

Modern research shows that royal jelly improves lipoprotein metabolism, promotes growth of neuronal stem cells and neurons, inhibits oxidation of lipids (as in brain tissue) and is a general antioxidant. A dose of 6 to 10 grams (6,000 to 10,000 mg) per day, essentially used in food quantities, is recommended.

Cocoa

Cocoa contains biologically active flavonols and polyphenols. Flavonols have recently been the subject of much research. They have been found to enhance vasodilation which in turn decreases blood pressure and increases peripheral blood flow to the muscles as well as to the brain. Cocoa has also been shown to improve lipid metabolism. And international researchers have recently uncovered even more healthy properties associated with the flavonol antioxidants found in cocoa beans.

Eighteen chocolate-centered studies—including investigations of how cocoa might affect blood pressure, heart disease, painful nerve disorders and cancer risk—were presented at the American Chemical Society's annual meeting in March 2012. These studies establish the biological plausibility of antioxidant effects of dark chocolate in small groups and even demonstrated the potential harm-reducing effects for smokers.

But don't look for health benefits from your favorite milk chocolate candy bar. Most of the studies used unsweetened regular cocoa powder. There are a couple of degrees of separation because when you make chocolate you add fat, in the form of cocoa butter and sugar. And nobody's going to eat a tablespoon of unsweetened cocoa. So the studies used cocoa-flavonoid compound supplements, with average doses of 400 to 500 milligrams. Which is equivalent to 32 bars of milk chocolate or eight to nine bars of dark chocolate. Too much for even the most die-hard chocoholic.

You can find cocoa flavonol extract supplements with up to 1,000 mg in natural supplement shops and from online supplement retailers.

Virgin Coconut Oil

Coconut oil, in its virgin state, is a tropical oil consisting of medium-chain fatty acids that convert readily into energy and are not stored in the body as fat. These kinds of essential fats are important for brain tissue cell membranes and neuronal sheaths.

A saturated fat, it has been maligned for several decades as a result of misinformation by the vegetable oil industry. Alternative health practitioners advocate coconut oil consumption for weight loss and maintenance regimens. Coconut oil is a rich source of lauric acid and monolaurin, known agents that are being explored by pharmaceutical companies for drug development potential. Coconut oil lowers lipoprotein cholesterol levels in the blood and tissues and lowers lipoprotein markers for heart attack.

A dosage of 20 grams (20,000 mg), essentially in food quantities, appears beneficial.

Taurine

Taurine is so named because it was initially isolated from ox bile (*Taurus, the bull*). It is a beta-amino acid gaining attention from researchers and supplement manufacturers for health-promoting and anti-aging properties.

Research has shown taurine plays a role in the function of skeletal muscles and the central nervous system, as well as regulating blood pressure and glucose levels. It's also being explored as an adaptogen and anti-anxiety agent. Taurine has been identified as an amino acid neurotransmitter.

A dose of 500 mg per day offers sufficient health benefits.

Lutein

Lutein is a prominent constituent of green, leafy vegetables. I helped discover its role in human metabolism and nutrition in the 1980's. Since then, it has developed a role in vision and eye health as a dietary supplement. Since the eye contains neurological tissue, this has led to current interest in its possible benefits for the brain. In addition to eating green leafy vegetables, a daily dose of 12 mg of lutein is recommended.

Going above and beyond for total protection

In addition to supplementation, staying active (mentally and physically) will help keep your brain fit as well as your body. Do the daily crossword puzzle and keep up with your monthly *Insiders' Cures* newsletter and *Daily Dispatch* emails.

A healthy diet and maintaining a healthy weight is also important (see Chapter 27). And controlling blood pressure and heart disease is key to maintaining healthy circulation and blood flow to the brain (and to avoiding strokes) (see Chapter 22). Controlling diabetes is also critical as high blood sugar can destroy nerves and the blood vessels that supply them.

Chapter 19

Vitamin E outperforms drug for Alzheimer's disease

All of the nutrients I've discussed so far are important for keeping your brain functioning as you age. But according to a new study, a simple vitamin may be the one of the biggest brain breakthroughs to come along in decades.

Researchers have found that people who have high levels of vitamin E tocotrienols in their blood have a lower risk of cognitive impairment—including Alzheimer's disease.

In fact, in a new study, men and women with AD who took this vitamin significantly delayed the progress of their disease. They lived longer overall.[6] Plus, perhaps more importantly, they lived longer *independently*.

Here's another interesting point about this study…

Researchers compared the vitamin to a drug commonly prescribed to treat moderate-to-severe AD patients. And the vitamin **outperformed** the drug!

For this study, published in the *Journal of the American Medical Association* (JAMA), researchers recruited 613 patients with mild-to-moderate Alzheimer's disease. Most of the participants attended 14 various Veteran's Affairs medical centers around the country. Researchers randomly divided them into four groups.

The first group took 2,000 IU of vitamin E each day for a little over two years, on average. Vitamin E is a fat-soluble vitamin that acts as an antioxidant. It can slow down processes that damage cells in the brain and elsewhere.

The second group took 20 mg of Memantine, a commonly prescribed AD drug. The third group took *both* vitamin E and Memantine. And the fourth group took a placebo.

Researchers found that the vitamin E group had significantly slower "functional" decline compared to the placebo group. This means they lived longer independently. They continued to do their own cooking, washing, and shopping. And they required less caregiver time and attention compared to the other three groups.

Overall, the researchers saw a "delay in clinical progression of 19 percent per year" in the vitamin E group compared to the placebo group.

Interestingly, neither the Memantine drug group nor the combined Memantine-vitamin E group showed any clinical benefits. Researchers think Memantine must interfere with how the body metabolizes vitamin E. It's a sad state of affairs, indeed, when a mainstream AD treatment not only doesn't work, but negates the effects of a basic nutrient that *does* work!

Vitamin E showed other benefits as well. The annual death rate in the vitamin E group was only 7.3 percent. But the groups that didn't take vitamin E had an annual death rate of 9.4 percent.

This study shows used a daily dose of 2,000 IU of natural mixed vitamin E. A level which has struck some awestruck observers as "high"—but only because RDA's are so ridiculously low to begin with.

Tocotrienols also appear to help <u>prevent</u> cancer (<u>including</u> prostate cancer), as well as cardiovascular disease.

All it takes is some real knowledge of human diet and nutrition to make sense of the isolated bits and pieces from today's often incoherent medical research.

Just don't look to the FDA or the mainstream government-industrial-medical complex to provide that knowledge or guidance.

My advice?

While we continue to wait for more useful results to come in, you can't go wrong taking 50 IU per day of vitamin E (as d-alpha tocopheryl acetate). If you are actually struggling with dementia, check with your doctor about upping your dose of vitamin E. Hopefully he or she is not still following the misguided, outdated research from 10 years ago.

Yes, in this study, Alzheimer's disease patients took 2,000 IU of vitamin E daily. And their symptoms improved. But remember, when you take a vitamin to <u>treat</u> a disease, it will most likely require much higher doses than when you take one for general health. Unfortunately, most researchers don't get this right when they study nutrients for chronic diseases. Instead, they use low-ball doses that can't reverse a disease that took a lifetime to develop.

But when you use vitamins primarily to support general health, you must consider many different factors, such as:

1. **How much of the nutrient do multivitamins or once-a-day vitamins contain?** When I make dosage recommendations for individual nutrients, such as vitamin E, I must consider that many people probably already take a daily multivitamin. And when recommending a specific dosage, I allow for the amount many already get in the daily multivitamin. In this case, typical multivitamins contain 100 IU of vitamin E. So, when I recommend taking 50 IU of vitamin E, it takes into account that many already get 100 IU from multivitamins.

2. **How much is the Daily Recommended Allowance?** I also consider the USDA's Daily Recommended Allowance (RDA). While RDA's are by no means the basis of my recommendations, and they are wholly inadequate for reversing chronic diseases, I certainly don't ignore the standard. In this case, the RDA for vitamin E is only 22 IU. However, the RDA goes on to state a "safe upper limit" of 1500 IU.

3. **How much of the nutrient can we assume an average healthy adult already gets through diet?** Remember, the purpose of dietary of supplements is to "supplement" what is already in your diet. For general health, your goal should be to get most of your nutrition from the whole foods you

eat. And I assume if you're interested in supplementing with vitamin E, you're also highly educated about good nutrition. And probably eating better than average to begin with. You also get large amounts of vitamin E by eating green, leafy vegetables, healthy oils, eggs, nuts, and seafood. So, when I recommend supplementing with vitamin E, I take these dietary sources of vitamin E into account.

4. **What other supplements do you take?** Manufacturers often add vitamin E to their "custom" supplements. So starting with 50 IU gives you room to get vitamin E from these other supplements as well as from dietary sources.

All things considered, 50 IU of vitamin E is a safe place to start for anyone and everyone who wants to support their general health. Now, as I said, if you want to treat a specific disease, like Alzheimer's disease, you will likely need a higher dose. But in that case, as with the management of any medical condition, a qualified doctor should closely supervise your regimen.

I often look with alarm at some of the dosages I see in typical, "run-of-the-mill" dietary supplements. It seems to me that much of the supplement industry just throws in "mega" doses and "super" doses. But they don't have any real science to support these excessive doses in the general population.

Maybe they think it looks more impressive. But *excess does not equal success*. That's just not how a healthy, balanced approach works.

My mentor, the late C. Everett Koop, former U.S. Surgeon General, used to quote, "the least medicine that works is the best medicine."

Let's keep working with the right doses, not just the largest.

In addition, make sure to get plenty of all the B vitamins. Folic acid is especially important. It helps reduce homocysteine levels, which sharply increase your risk of developing AD and heart disease. In one European study, a daily dose of 800 micrograms of folic acid significantly lowered homocysteine. It also improved cognitive function and memory in middle-aged and older adults.

Chapter 20

Profits—not cures—for Alzheimer's disease

Over 20 years ago, I attended a big government event in Washington, D.C. where science bureaucrats announced the "Decade of the Brain." At the event, they claimed we would conquer brain and neurological diseases over the next 10 years. And they proudly proclaimed massive increases in spending on research for brain and nervous system illnesses.

But clearly, it was just a publicity stunt to get more new funding from the taxpayers for more of the same old research.

During that "Decade of the Brain," science made little—if any—real headway regarding treatments. Instead, we endured 10 years of disappointing clinical drug trials, with virtually no progress toward curing or preventing brain diseases.

In February of 2014, the Obama administration announced another "Decade of the Brain." But here again, it's just a publicity stunt to spend more of your tax dollars.

Of course, brain changes can occur 10 to 20 years before you experience any overt symptoms of AD. So, by the time doctors diagnose you with dementia, too much damage has already occurred.

So early prevention not only makes sense...it's critical.

But government health officials and mainstream medicine continue to ignore berberine and vitamin E as viable AD treatments. They also ignore the apparent risk of lowering cholesterol levels for the brain. And they certainly don't give credit to the role vitamin D and B complex play in protecting cognition and neurological function.

They simply want you to take "new" drugs to prevent a disease they can't treat.

So, what are some of the new drug approaches proposed to prevent dementia? And, do they present opportunities for *true* prevention?

One approach targets the formation of a protein called beta-amyloid. In AD patients, this protein clumps into plaques in the brain. It disrupts the flow of information across nerve synapses and causes nerve cell death. But—unlike vitamin E—these drugs fail to stop the progress of AD.

So now, they're trying the failed beta-amyloid drugs out as "preventative" drugs. They can then give these failed drugs to younger people, before they present with AD symptoms. Just look at what's happening in Yarumal, Columbia…

In this small town, men and women get AD in their late 40s--about 15 years ahead of the norm. Researchers discovered they carry a gene variant associated with early-onset dementia.

In a clinical trial that began in 2013, men and women in their 30s from this small town who carry the gene began taking a drug developed by Genentech. Researchers hope the drug will prevent AD by blocking or slowing the formation of beta-amyloid plaques in the brain.

Since people with this gene form beta-amyloid earlier in life, anti-amyloid drugs are supposed to help in this genetic form. I worry if the study shows even a glimmer of promise, doctors will one day begin doling out AD drugs to anyone like candy to "prevent" AD. Like they do now with statin drugs, with their claim to "prevent" cardiovascular disease.

And the consequences could be just as deadly.

Fortunately, with the information you've just read, you're

armed with real, scientifically proven cures. Ones that can keep you and your loved ones from suffering the devastating effects of Alzheimer's and other forms of dementia.

MASTER YOUR HEART HEALTH

Part 4: Master your heart health

Chapter 21
Shocking results! Not all is as it seems

In 1976, I was among a small group of U.S. graduate students awarded a scholarship to study in Asia. The scholarship was awarded by the Henry Luce Foundation (Founder of *Time*, *Life*, and *Fortune* magazines—who had been born in China of U.S. missionaries). Though it was barely one year after the last of the Americans were evacuated by helicopter from the rooftop of the U.S. Embassy in Saigon, Vietnam, I decided to conduct my studies in Southeast Asia.

Unlike the other scholars who landed in large urban areas (what demographers call "primate" cities, like Taipei, Bangkok, Jakarta, Singapore, and Manila) I chose to go into the jungles of Mindanao, Philippines, bordering on the Spice Islands of storied history. There, I sought a more authentic encounter with indigenous cultures.

I went to an area called, *"Donde Non Hay Doctor,"* or "where there is no doctor." These tens of thousands of islands, as well as the Malayan Peninsula, of Southeast Asia make up a living archaeology of human settlements. The original peoples of the area were pushed into the deep interior of the jungle islands by the arrival thousands of years ago by the Malay peoples of today. During the ancient era, the expansion of Hindu culture, Chinese mercantile influences, and the expansion of Islam turned Southeast Asia into the perfect melting pot to observe traditional healing. Including shamans, herbalists, midwives, and other traditional healers. Pretty good for a place that claims to have no doctor...

My base in Davao represented a rapidly growing population. It was quickly moving from a rural to urban setting, resulting in conflicts among the many different cultures and languages of Southeast Asia. In this environment, school children were rigorously segregated according to their abilities in performance in school.

My goal was to establish standards for normal blood pressure in children. All we knew at that time is that blood pressure is low (and heart rate high) in younger children and blood pressure increases as children age, until reaching the "normal" blood pressure of adulthood, which we say is 120/80.

I gathered the data, class by class. And soon, a pattern became clear. The rate of "higher" blood pressure was much greater among the remedial students in each grade, in each age group. So the students who did poorly in school were the ones with higher blood pressure.

So I started to look for physiological causes for the high blood pressure. Something that might be making the children "sick," that might account for their poor performance in school. But I couldn't figure it out. I couldn't find any physiological reason for these children to have high blood pressure. Nor a connection to their poor performance.

When I returned to the U.S., I mentioned my conundrum to a friend of mine, a neighbor of my parents. He was the Chairman of Physiology at the University of California and an expert on environmental physiology and stress. He was running studies in the "space age" Human Centrifuge Laboratory where they exposed humans to high stress and measured the effects of stress on raising blood pressure. And he was quick to point out the error in my thinking. When I turned my analysis around, I realized that the increased stress of doing poorly in school, and being segregated and treated poorly by the teachers, was responsible for raising blood pressure in these poor students.

Now, it's important to note that back then, "modern" medicine gave very little credence to the role of stress in health (just as it ignored nutrition). So my theory was debated.

Some had suggested that the students with high blood pressure must be drinking water with more salt in it. But the body is normally able to remove excess salt unless there is a reason for it to hang on to excess fluid and electrolytes (like salt). This can happen in times of stress. And, in Southeast Asia, there were traditional fishing villages that had the highest intake of salt yet recorded... yet blood pressure was actually low in adults and the elderly. Only when those villages were disrupted and the fishing communities moved from rural to urban areas, did blood pressure levels rapidly increase in those displaced and stressed populations.

So I persisted in defending my conclusion that stress was actually the cause of the high blood pressure. And finally, I was able to publish my results, as a student, in the *American Journal of Public Health*.

Fortunately times have changed. And my research prevailed. Today, nearly everyone understands how important stress can be to blood pressure and cardiovascular disease. The problem now, however, is how overlooked—or perhaps I should say "overshadowed"—blood pressure is as a primary risk factor for heart disease.

Cholesterol is NOT the most important risk factor for heart disease

A lavish amount of attention, effort, and money has been spent on controlling cholesterol. And the great medical-pharmaceutical complex has worked relentlessly to continue to lower the recommended cholesterol level for heart health. Of course, the end result is that more and more people will be caught in the net of taking dangerous cholesterol-lowering drugs.

But the truth is...half of the people who die of heart disease have *normal* cholesterol levels. And lowering cholesterol by a few points may not have any effect at all. Cholesterol is NOT the most important risk factor it's set up to be.

Blood pressure, on the other hand, is a *much* different story. Above all else, controlling blood pressure has the most direct and essential connection to cutting heart disease. The importance of controlling blood pressure should not be overlooked, or taken for granted. While lowering cholesterol by a few points may or may not have any benefit, lowering blood pressure by even a few points is *always* worthwhile.

And when it comes to your heart's greatest threat, I have what might be a *surprising* recommendation...

Seven critical heart health markers more important than cholesterol

Doctors routinely measure fasting blood glucose and insulin levels as well as hemoglobin A1C in people with diabetes. The first two of these tests are well known, but you may not be as familiar with hemoglobin A1C. This test gives a good long-term measure of your average blood sugar numbers over time.

Unfortunately, many doctors still don't measure homocysteine levels and do not take them seriously. But they should. Your body uses homocysteine to make protein and to build and maintain tissue. However, too much of this substance may increase your risk of stroke, certain types of heart disease, and peripheral artery disease.

So, without further ado, here are the targets for these four critical heart disease markers.

Fasting blood glucose. The ideal range is 65 to 99 mg/dL. However, if your hemoglobin A1C is at a healthy, lower level, your doctor will likely be less concerned if your blood glucose is over 99 in a single test.

Fasting insulin. A normal level is below 5 uIU/mL, but ideally you'll want it below 3.

Hemoglobin A1C should be between 4.4 and 6.5 percent.

Homocysteine. The Mayo Clinic says a normal level is between 4.4 and 10.8 µmol/L.[1]

To help get all of these numbers where you want them, focus on improving your diet. (See Part 5 of this book for more on diet and proper hydration)

But there are a few more important factors to consider in assessing your overall heart health. And, unfortunately, your doctor is even less likely to monitor these markers. Unless, of course, you insist on it.

Three more heart health markers you should keep close tabs on

Other important measurements you should consider are C-reactive protein (CRP) and fibrinogen. CRP is a marker of inflammation. Research has linked CRP to increased risk of coronary artery disease. And fibrinogen is a protein involved in blood clotting. Elevated levels can lead to dangerous artery-blocking clots.

Combined with the other parameters I mentioned above, these tests can help your doctor assess your overall risk of heart disease.

Your CRP level should be less than 1 mg/L, and your fibrinogen level should be between 200 and 400 mg/dL. To achieve this, follow a healthy, balanced diet. High-quality fish oils are particularly helpful at reducing the chronic inflammation that can boost your CRP level.

And keep in mind that research is also showing that your vitamin D level may be just as important as other tests in determining your risk of heart disease. A blood level above 50 ng/ml is healthy, and a daily dose of 4,000 to 5,000 IU of vitamin D is safe and appropriate for everyone.

One final heart-healthy tip: Avoid excess iron. It can potentially accumulate in your heart muscle and other tissues, eventually leading to organ failure in some people. I've also conducted research with Nobel laureate Baruch Blumberg that showed that excess iron in the body increases the risk of cancer in both men and women.[2] Never take a supplement containing iron unless you have been diagnosed by a doctor with an iron deficiency.

Chapter 22

The ONE prescription I will *always* recommend for high blood pressure

This powerful cause of heart disease requires a potent remedy.

Admittedly, one of the challenges of natural, alternative therapies is that, while effective, they are gentler and generally take effect over longer periods of time as compared to their highly-potent drug counterparts. And when it comes to lowering high blood pressure, you need to use something that is going to work fast.

Extremists who reject ALL drugs in favor of natural supplements have nothing to talk about here, because there aren't really any dietary supplements that can bring down high blood pressure quickly. While some "natural experts" may claim to have nutrients that work for supporting blood pressure...don't be fooled.

There are many that can support heart health overall, which I will show you in Chapter 25, but none will compare to the most effective, and necessary approach—taking a blood pressure medication.

So, while there are many natural medicine "experts" who won't—or can't—recommend a drug medication, I can and will when it is the best medicine.

While there *are* many effective "mind-body" therapies that can help manage your underlying stress there is no acceptable alternative treatment that can substitute for fast and effective drug therapy for this dangerous condition. And fortunately, modern medicine has developed many safe and effective drugs to control blood pressure over the decades.

If you have high blood pressure you should have your blood pressure monitored and treated by a physician using these effective drug therapies. However, you and your doctor need not run to the latest, most expensive blood pressure drug offered by the drug industry. It is important to choose wisely.

What to look for...

Safe and effective drugs for blood pressure have been around for several decades with an immense amount of clinical experience on their best uses. Many people don't realize that even after a new drug is "approved" for use by the FDA, something called "post-marketing surveillance" is required to continue for many years.

It is during this surveillance, when drugs are being used by millions of people over many years, that so many of the disastrous side effects of many drugs are discovered. This is why we are constantly hearing that new drugs "approved" by the FDA are found to have dangerous side effects and the FDA issues "warnings" and restrictions, or they are pulled off the market altogether.

So when it comes to choosing a blood pressure drug, the safest course of action is to work with your doctor to choose one that's been around for many years. This could also save you a lot of money, since you'll have more generic drugs to choose from, which are a fraction of the cost of new, still-patented drugs. The point is—newer is not always better—or safer. Especially when it comes to anti-hypertensive medications.

Talk to your physician about trying out these older, effective drugs for controlling blood pressure. Remember, everyone is an individual and may react differently to different medications. It may take some trial and error, with very close monitoring, to find the right medication for you.

The older drugs for blood pressure fall under the following categories:

1. Drugs that act to lower blood pressure through their effect on the nervous system

Clonidine   Reserpine
Methyldopa   Propranolol

2. Drugs that lower blood pressure by their effect on nerve endings

> Guanethidine
> Monoamine oxidase inhibitors
> Reserpine

3. Drugs that lower blood pressure by dilating blood vessels

> Diazoxide   Nitroprusside
> Hydralazine   Prazosin
> Minoxidil   Thiazides

4. Drugs that lower blood pressure by blocking nerve receptors ("Beta" and "Alpha" Blockers)

> Metapropolol   Phenoxybenzamine
> Nadolol   Prazosin
> Phentolamine   Propranolol

5. Drugs that lower blood pressure by influencing blood-pressure regulating hormones produced by the kidney

> Captopril
> Saralasin

These drugs are given by their generic names as they are all off patent. Check with your doctor to see what is available by prescription and if they are appropriate for you.

Survival guide to blood pressure medications

Believe it or not, 100 years ago, blood pressure medicines contained cyanide. Not surprisingly, they caused some thoroughly unpleasant side effects. So it was often hard to get patients to stay on these medications. Unlike most drugs that address the symptoms of a disease, patients felt better when they stopped the medications.

Luckily, in more recent decades better, safer, more effective drugs have become available. There are still a few potential side effects. But in most cases, they're easily managed.

Beta-Blockers (like Propranolol) block adrenalin, relax and open the blood vessels for easier flow, and can reduce the speed and force of the heartbeat. But because they block adrenalin, they also can cause side effects such as faintness, dizziness, and cold extremities. They can also narrow the air passages in the lungs, which may cause wheezing, cough, and shortness of breath. Alpha-blockers are somewhat similar but may also increase cholesterol and weight gain, as well as episodes of sudden drops in blood pressure.

If you suffer any of these side effects, see your doctor about adjusting the dose or the prescription. And remember to ask about drugs that are "off patent." They're less expensive and have stood the test of time in establishing their safety.

Diuretics (or "water pills") are designed to eliminate excess fluids, making it easier for the heart to pump. They increase urination, which may already be a problem in men with prostate problems. And it may also allow key nutrients to escape in the extra urine. Most physicians recognize the potential loss of potassium, but may not be aware of the loss of other nutrients.

If you're taking a diuretic, make sure you are well hydrated and have adequate intake of vitamins and minerals.

Vasodilators relax and open the blood vessels, which allows blood to flow more freely and reduces blood pressure. However, they may cause problems similar to the ones listed above for Beta-Blockers.

Some of these potential symptoms may have you raising your eyebrows. But rest assured, if there's one thing modern medicine is good at it is managing diseases with drugs. And also managing the well-known and accepted side effects of those drugs. And in the case of high blood pressure, the benefit of swiftly and efficiently lowering it with the use of drugs far outweighs the risks of the side effects of the drugs.

But, again, one of the easiest ways you can help control the costs and the side effects of blood pressure medications is to consult your doctor about using a "generic." These have been around long enough to go "off patent," which dramatically lowers the price. And they've been used long enough that the FDA has had a chance to discover any hidden problems that emerged after they "approved" the drug. Which means your doctor will be well-equipped to spot—and deal with—any potential side effects that may occur. Some of these older drugs include Diazoxide, Hydralazine, Minoxidil, Nitroprusside, Prazosin, and Thiazides.

And, of course, it's just as important with high blood pressure as it is with any chronic condition to adopt a healthy diet and exercise program, lose weight, and reduce or manage stress through any number of effective "mind-body" techniques.

8 easy steps to soothe stress right now

In the meantime, you can get started now towards any mind-body approach to managing stress by following these eight easy steps...

1. Pick a word or short phrase that has personal meaning, such as "love" or "peace," or the Christian "Lord is my shepherd," or Jewish "shalom"

2. Sit quietly in a comfortable position

3. Close your eyes

4. Relax your muscles

5. Breathe slowly, naturally, repeating your word or phrase silently, as you exhale

6. Take a passive attitude, dismiss all distractions

7. Continue for 10 to 12 minutes; do not stand for another 1 or 2 minutes

8. Repeat twice per day

Chapter 23

Starting NOW—Heart healthy relaxation tactics from the "Inside"

Once you have your blood pressure under control through appropriate drug therapy and monitoring by a physician, it is time to address the underlying stress that contributes to high blood pressure, heart disease, and many if not most other chronic diseases.

A basic approach in all of natural medicine is that the mind and body work together and each continually influences the other. Thus, nearly any effective therapy is essentially a mind-body therapy. However, some therapies are specifically called "mind-body" because they appear to draw directly on the power of our thoughts, emotions, and feelings to influence the disease or healthy states of our normal body functions. Literally, "mind over matter." There are several that are safe, proven effective, and widely available.

Biofeedback. We all learn as adults to control our emotions and feelings and to project a calm and controlled image to the outside world. But under the rigid exterior of the body, our feelings have a torrent of effects on our internal workings. Biofeedback gives us back information about how blood pressure, heart rate, and other vital signs are responding to environmental stimuli and stresses—and teaches how to consciously control our reactions for a healthier, stress-free response to life.

Guided Imagery. Visualization is a powerful ability the mind. You can literally create images in your "mind's eye" and train yourself to see your body becoming healthier. You can visualize a picture of immune system cells destroying cancer cells, for example. Or you can imagine yourself in a calm, healing environment and literally take your body to that place physiologically, lowering your blood pressure along the way.

Hypnosis. Today, hypnosis is understood as using the "power of suggestion" to move mind-body connections in proper alignment for healthier outcomes.

Meditation & Yoga. There are different approaches to meditation. Transcendental Meditation (TM) came to the U.S. from India, but there are strong traditions of meditation, or "contemplative thought," in the early U.S., dating from our Founding Fathers, such as Adams and Jefferson, to men of American letters, such as Emerson and Thoreau. And today, it can be seen as a simple, practical "break" from our hectic day. We can think of this form as Mindfulness Meditation. Simply paying attention to what is happening in the moment and how you are feeling about it.

Likewise, yoga is used to enter meditative states. There are several approaches in India but the Hatha-Yoga tradition, emphasizing physical postures and breathing, has become most popular in the west (probably because of its emphasis on the physical vs. mental aspects of meditation). Either way, yoga and meditation are pathways to the mind-body connection whereby entering into a more peaceful, calm state has clear benefits in lowering blood pressure and improving health.

These are just a few of the prominent mind-body techniques that are available. Though keep in mind, not all of these techniques will work for everyone. To find out which will work best for you, take the "Find Your Boundary Type" quiz on my website, www. drmicozzi.com.

Chapter 24

Heal your heart with what you eat and *how* you eat it

As you can see, you can control blood pressure with appropriate drug medications and reduce stress with effective mind-body techniques. These are important steps to reducing heart disease and promoting heart health.

But preventing the development of heart disease is an area where diet and nutrition, alternative treatments, and dietary supplements also have an important role. The body is not static—it has the ability to heal itself. This is an important basis of all alternative and complementary remedies, whether they are dietary supplements and herbs, or mind-body techniques.

In fact, my colleague, Dr. Dean Ornish (who co-chaired my medical conference on Complementary & Alternative Medicine in 1999) has shown the right diet can not only prevent but actually reverse heart disease.

Dr. Ornish emphasizes the benefits of the low-fat, high-carbohydrate aspect of his diet. Unfortunately, I think some of his recommendations are downright wrong. I'll discuss those in just a moment. But first, there is one aspect to the Ornish plan that I do agree with. He recommends that participants ideally eat together, and even cook and shop for food together. This provides much-needed social support and positive interaction with other motivated people.

Human diet is a behavior. People eat foods not nutrients. And the way we eat may be just as important as what we eat. Chinese Medicine and Ayurveda stress the way we eat: They place emphasis on the time of day, food and beverage combinations, family and social and community circumstances, even the seasons of the year. These are all aspects that are completely ignored by mainstream medicine and the natural products industry alike.

Fifteen years ago, epidemiologists puzzled over the "French Paradox"—that is, the French eat the "wrong" things in their diet (like cheese, liver pate, and pastries), smoke more, and drink more wine, on average—but their rate of heart disease is half that in the U.S.!

The epidemiologists did not know to take into account the traditional French lifestyle of taking two hours for lunch (often adding a little nap time). They eat slowly and in social circumstances, insisting on fresh and deliciously prepared dishes. And they take six or eight weeks off for the summer, with frequent long, three- and four-day weekends and holidays in between. The epidemiologists also did not understand the stress-reducing benefits of moderate wine consumption.

We had our own example of the French paradox here in the U.S. in the little Italian-American community of Rosetto, Pennsylvania. Residents here ate too much of the wrong foods, drank more wine, and smoked more—but were healthier. It turns out they were happy, had strong families, loved their neighbors and cared about their community. A little bit of kindness and love goes a long way for the "heart."

Our bodies are not defenseless when it comes to metabolizing rich foods, alcohol, or even tobacco smoke. A positive mindset and healthy habits of how we eat are just as important as what we eat.

And in terms of what we eat, when it comes to heart health, no two foods have been vilified more than salt and fat.

But do they really deserve their bad reputations?

The great salt scam

One of the wonders of the great American west is the Great Salt Lake. But today's informed physicians and scientists are wondering about "The Great Salt Scam." Promulgated, of course, by none other than the federal government.

For years we've labored under bad science when it comes to salt and blood pressure.

We've been fed a steady diet of misinformation that salt raises blood pressure, causes hypertension, and can lead to premature death.

But the fact is, if you have healthy kidneys, your body should be able to get rid of any excess salt. Subject those kidneys to a huge amount of stress however, and you may have problems.

Although it should be a settled issue by now, the great "war" against salt continues to rage even today. (Probably because the war helps keep a lot of political scientists and science bureaucrats employed working in the "salt mines.")

One anti-salt apostle even claims, "salt is the new tobacco." But this is an unscientific opinion. And it's not even half-right.

As you know, the U.S. government has made salt a public enemy for one main reason…

They claim it causes high blood pressure.

As I always say, *stress* is the No. 1 cause of high blood pressure in most people. And salt is only a primary problem for a small minority.

But the government treats us all the same. And it treats salt like a villain, with a "zero-tolerance" policy.

They recommend you limit salt intake to no more than 2,300 mg per day.

But this limit is ridiculous. Fewer than one-one hundredth of one percent (0.01 percent) of the population can achieve the government guideline. Plus, it's unhealthy–and lacks a fundamental understanding of human biology.

You see, sodium is an essential mineral. Your body needs it for all cellular communications, hydration, and essential physiologic functions. We should all make sure to get enough fluid and electrolytes. And what is *the* major electrolyte in the body? Sodium.

So your real goal should be to achieve balance. Not a nearly zero salt intake.

In fact, the optimal range for salt intake falls between 3,000 mg and 6,000 mg per day. That's 3 to 6 grams. (In terms of the government's "war on salt," we can think of this range as the "demilitarized" zone.)

In fact, a new study confirms my view...

Researchers recently conducted a new analysis of the PURE Study (Prospective Urban-Rural Epidemiology). They looked at data for 101,945 participants and found that men and women who consumed 3,000 to 6,000 mg of sodium per day had the lowest risk of cardiovascular disease events and deaths. But when patients went outside that zone, they landed in a salt pile of trouble.

Researchers found that men and women with either high or low sodium intake increased their cardiovascular disease risk. And this connection held up among people with and without high blood pressure.

Of course, the low-salt warriors immediately attacked these findings. They say the study's findings challenge the American Heart Association's (AHA) recommendations. (How dare the facts challenge the dogma?)

Like the U.S. government, the AHA says everyone should keep their sodium intake below 2,300 mg of sodium per day. Plus, if you're over age 51 years and/or African-American, the AHA says you should limit yourself to 1,500 mg of sodium per day.

That's half the lower limit of the PURE study's "safety zone." And it puts millions of Americans at risk!

You see, in the PURE analysis, the average sodium intake was 4,900 mg per day. According to the AHA, with numbers like those, everyone in the study should be dropping like flies. But only 8 percent actually had cardiovascular disease!

Overall, about half of the participants consumed between 4,000 and 6,000 mg sodium daily. Only 10 percent of participants consumed less than 3,000 mg per day. And nobody consumed less than 2,300 mg (the government and the AHA's ridiculous "maximum" limit).

But those who consumed less than 3,000 mg per day actually had a 25 percent increased risk of cardiovascular events *and* all-cause mortality! So, clearly the AHA's guidelines place everyone at risk of higher death rates and cardiovascular events.

Of course, it's important to note that there is a safety zone. And there *may* be such a thing as too much salt.

At the very highest end, men and women who consumed more than 7,000 mg of sodium per day had a 15 percent increased risk of death and cardiovascular events. (But remember, the low-salt group's risk went up by 25 percent!)

Now—let's look at the numbers for men and women in the study who did not have high blood pressure...

The low-salt group with normal blood pressure had an increased risk of cardiovascular events and death. But the high-salt group with normal blood pressure had no increased risk at all. So this confirms that the real problem is high blood pressure, not high salt. Or, put another way, these findings show that unless you have high blood pressure, there is no reason to worry about salt.

These results may surprise you. But they shouldn't. The PURE study isn't a lone shot in the dark. This kind of data has been around for a long time.

Data from two other major studies—the ONTARGET and TRANSCEND studies—support the PURE study results. Together, these two other studies followed 28,880 men and women at higher risk of cardiovascular disease. In these studies, men and women who consumed less than 3,000 mg sodium per day had an increased risk of suffering a cardiovascular event, such as a heart attack or stroke.

So, once again, the U.S. government and the AHA have been giving us bad advice all along. But real science shows you don't need to worry about salt (especially if you have normal blood pressure) except to make sure you're getting enough.

And while we're on the topic of bad advice, let's talk about another food you've been told to cut back on in the name of heart health...

Three big fat myths still being mouthed by "experts"

"Fat and cholesterol are bad." How often have you heard that? Even though these innocent nutrients are so essential that we literally could not live without them, we're still barraged every day by old myths and misconceptions promulgated by fat phobics and cholesterol cholerics.

Even worse, these myths continue to come straight from the mouths of paid experts who really should know better by now.

It is astounding to me that decades-old, ill-informed comments and recommendations about fat and cholesterol are still being made today. Despite the lack of any real proof—and a bunch of evidence to the contrary.

Here's a look at three commonly repeated fat and cholesterol "facts" that are as mythical as the nine lives of a cat.

Myth 1:
You'll have a heart attack if you eat saturated fat

The idea that saturated fat raises the risk of heart disease was initially based on flawed studies that clueless politicians, abetted by political scientists, somehow made into public policy.

The saturated fat myth is based on a chain of misconceptions. We've since learned that consuming saturated fat does not really appear to raise LDL "bad" cholesterol by much[3,4] (Even assuming that cholesterol is the culprit behind heart disease in the first place—see Myth 6).

Saturated fat actually appears to change LDL from small, dense particles that can clog arteries to larger, lighter particles that are mostly benign.[5] Further, saturated fat appears to raise HDL "good" cholesterol.

So, if anything, saturated fat seems to actually *improve* cholesterol profile in terms of supposed heart disease risk factors.

Still not convinced? Consider this: In 2010, researchers reviewed data from 21 studies involving 347,747 participants and found no evidence that saturated fat consumption increases the risk of heart disease.[6]

You can't get much more proof than that.

Myth 2:
Foods that contain cholesterol will kill you

Cholesterol in food is broken down during digestion and has no correlation to the cholesterol that circulates in the blood. Nor does dietary cholesterol intake correlate to heart disease.

I repeat: Cholesterol in food is not the same as the cholesterol we've all been taught (misguidedly) to fear.

This tragic lack of basic knowledge and understanding has led to excellent, healthy foods such as eggs, lobster, and shrimp being consigned to the "bad list" simply because they contain cholesterol. To this day, so-called experts still drone on about how many eggs or shellfish servings you can "get away with."

There is nothing wrong with eating shellfish if you enjoy it. And eggs are actually nature's perfect food, packed with minerals, vitamins, and other nutrients. But keep in mind these nutrients are found in the yolk, which is also the part of the egg that contains cholesterol. Advising people to throw out the yolks and only eat egg whites is just about the most ridiculous and wasteful advice in the sad history of diet and nutrition recommendations.

Myth 3:
LDL cholesterol is evil

Mainstream medicine is obsessed with lowering total and LDL "bad" cholesterol in the blood. But while cardiologists drop the LDL limit ever lower, endocrinology doctors who are experts in human metabolism are crying foul.

Studies have found that total and LDL cholesterol levels are poor indicators of heart disease compared with other risk markers.[7]

I also recently reported on a study of 231,986 patients hospitalized for heart disease. Half of them had normal LDL cholesterol levels.[8]

And in older people, there are studies that show that the higher the cholesterol, the *lower* the risk of heart disease.[9]

My late colleague, Dr. Arthur Schatzkin of the National Cancer Institute, first showed that low cholesterol is a risk factor for cancer nearly 30 years ago. Recent studies have found low cholesterol is associated with higher mortality worldwide—not only from cancer, but also suicide.[10]

Despite all the research showing that these myths are nothing more than fairy tales that haven't come true, I continue to see warnings from nutritional "experts" about the evils of fat and cholesterol.

But now you know better. Just say no to these outrageous misconceptions that have been promulgated upon the American people over the last four decades. Your body will thank you.

Chapter 25

The Heart Disease Battle Plan:
Nine proven secrets for gaining control

As I mentioned above, there are many nutritional supplements that can benefit overall heart health. Following are nine of my favorites. These nutrients have been shown to help lower cholesterol, support the heart muscle, and promote free-flowing blood to the heart and circulation.

1. **Gugulipid.** Gugulipid, or gum-guggul, is from the resin of one of the remarkable gum trees found in South Asia,

Southeast Asia, and Australia. Centuries ago, gum tree resins were employed in the ancient Ayurvedic pharmacy. The knowledge of how and when to harvest the resins, how to prepare and store them, and how to administer them are critical to achieving its therapeutic benefits. There are accordingly questions about the supply, formulation, and potency of different preparations, so check with your qualified health practitioner about the sources and uses of this dietary supplement. But when used appropriately, this therapy has been shown to lower cholesterol.

2. **Garlic.** The clinical studies of garlic on heart health address three areas: (1) lipids, like cholesterol (2) blood pressure, and (3) atherosclerosis and thrombosis. Investigators have explored its use as a treatment for mild hypertension and high cholesterol. Heavy consumption may lead to slowed blood clotting, perioperative bleeding, and spontaneous hemorrhage. Numerous studies have long documented garlic's irreversible inhibitory effect on platelet aggregation and fibrinolytic activity in humans, which makes the blood "thinner."

To benefit from the heart health effects of garlic take one or two fresh cloves per day; or if using a garlic extract, take 200-400 mg, two to three times per day.

3. **B Vitamin and Flavonoids.** The levels of a chemical called homocysteine in the blood are strongly and consistently linked to the risk of heart disease. The leading researcher who has worked for decades to demonstrate this effect lives in my home town in New England. I brought him to speak to the College of Physicians in Philadelphia over 10 years ago to try to get the word out about this critically important finding. All these years later, your doctor may *still* not know to do anything about homocysteine. But lowering homocysteine to healthy levels is easily achieved by supplementing with folic acid, vitamin B6, and vitamin B12.

Try daily doses of 800 mcg of folic acid, 25-50 mg of vitamin B6, and 100-300 mcg of vitamin B 12.

4. **Selenium & Vitamin E.** Since selenium comes from the soil in which foods are grown, and livestock are grazed, selenium levels in the body often correlate. I studied the role of selenium in preventing cancer in China during the 1980's. But selenium is also important for the heart. Deep in the interior of Mainland China lies the land with the lowest levels of selenium anywhere on earth. In this low-selenium area of China, we find high rates of "Ke-Shan" disease, a deadly cardiomyopathy wherein the heart muscle itself does not function. Besides contributing to the health of the heart muscle, selenium also helps activate the important antioxidant enzyme, glutathione peroxidase, which is also important to heart health.

Selenium is often thought to work in combination with vitamin E, especially as an antioxidant. On its own, vitamin E protects low-density lipoprotein cholesterol from being oxidized and reduces heart disease.

Take selenium 100 mcg per day, and vitamin E 50 IU per day.

5. **Magnesium.** Magnesium deficiency can develop if you already have heart disease and are being treated for heart disease, especially with the use of digitalis and certain diuretic drugs. Some researchers believe that magnesium supplementation helps prevent the occurrence of sudden death in people with heart disease and helps increase survival.

Take 300-400 mg of magnesium per day for six weeks to restore healthy magnesium levels.

6. **Hawthorn.** Hawthorn is a member of the rose family with sharp thorns and small white or pink flowers that develop a bright red fruit, found in woodlands. The constituents improve heart muscle function, heart output, and blood flow in the coronary arteries and to the heart muscle. It also reduces resistance to blood flow.

Try a commonly used extract from leaves and flowers

standardized on total flavonoid or procyanidin content, 160-900 mg per day for 4 to 8 weeks. If using a traditional preparation of the berries or fruit, try 4 -5 grams per day.

7. **Terminalia arjuna.** This Ayurvedic herb has been well known in India for its heart benefits since at least 500 BC. It contains a flavone called arjunolone, as well as arjunic acid, and arjunetin and arjunosides, which are glycosides (like the better-known digitalis). Arjuna seems similar to other heart-active medicinal plants like Lilly of the Valley (*Convallaria majalis*) that help survival with heart disease. As with gugulipid, check with your health practitioner about appropriate sources and uses of this dietary supplement.

8. **Coenzyme Q10.** This critical enzyme co-factor is an essential component of mitochondrial membranes which are not only the energy factories of the cells but also produce water for proper hydration at the cell level (see *The Insider's answer to healthy aging and vitality*). The more active a cell needs to be in the body, the more immediate and important are its effects. The muscles do a lot of physical work, and especially the heart muscle. That's why drugs and chemicals that poison the mitochondria are so toxic to the heart and muscles as well as the other tissues and organs of the body. Coenzyme Q10 is coming to be considered a key nutritional supplement.

Try 30-50 mg of coenzyme Q10 per day.

9. **Red Yeast Rice.** Despite the hype and scare tactics that have surrounded it in recent years, red yeast rice remains a safe and effective option for lowering cholesterol levels. When choosing a red yeast rice product, look for four important things:

1. Choose organic.

2. Choose a product that has been processed to remove a potential toxin called citrinin, a by-product of the red yeast rice fermentation process.

3. Choose a supplement made in the USA that meets FDA Good Manufacturing Practices (GMPs) and the standards of US Pharmacopeia (USP).

4. Make sure it contains 1,200 mg of pure red yeast rice. Anything less and you will not be taking a clinically effective dose.

Red yeast rice can be combined with complementary ingredients to boost its effectiveness. Of course, as you now know, lowering your cholesterol is not enough for heart health. A more comprehensive approach is the best long-term solution.

A combined approach represents the best of complementary medicine: safe and effective drugs to control blood pressure, dietary supplements for heart health, a sensible program of diet and exercise, achieving and maintaining a healthy weight, and using effective mind-body therapies that match your emotional type for stress management.

10. **Vitamin D.** A new study from Germany highlights the heart benefits of the critical nutrient Vitamin D, which has so many healthy properties. Researchers found that vitamin D (a critical nutrient, deficiency of which is reaching worldwide "epidemic" levels) is associated with lower death rates in patients with heart disease, and overall. These researchers measured actual levels of vitamin D in the blood, rather than looking at daily intake of vitamin D.

Taking 1,000-2,000 IU of vitamin D is appropriate for most people.

Prevent heart disease with this key vitamin

New research shows older men and women who have adequate blood levels of vitamin D have lower cardiovascular disease risk.

You probably know the visible effects of inflammation–pain, redness, heat, and swelling. And you've probably experienced it after twisting an ankle or straining your back. In these cases, the inflammatory process is the first step toward self-healing.

But not all inflammation is the same. Some inflammation occurs inside the body–and it does not lead to healing. It only leads to destruction. In fact, inflammation in your cardiovascular system can cause damage to your heart and blood vessels.

So, as I've mentioned, it's very important to ask your doctor for the C-reactive protein (CRP) test.

If your numbers are too high, it means you have a lot of harmful inflammation in your cardiovascular system. And, therefore, you have a much higher risk of developing heart disease.

In a new study, researchers explored the role of vitamin D in inflammation and chronic disease in 957 healthy, older adults.[11,12] At the study's outset, the researchers measured the participants' vitamin D levels. They defined anything above 75 nmol/L as "sufficient" vitamin D. And anything below 25 nmol/L as "deficient."

They found that men and women *deficient* in vitamin D had higher levels of biomarkers linked with cardiovascular disease. In fact, they had significantly higher levels of C-reactive protein and interleukin-6 (another marker of inflammation tied to heart disease) compared to those who had sufficient vitamin D levels. The men and women were also more likely to have other inflammatory conditions, such as multiple sclerosis (MS) and rheumatoid arthritis.

In an interview, Dr. Clifford J. Rosen of Tufts University School of Medicine underscored the importance of this study. He said, "I think all of us now think that inflammation is a critical factor in a lot of disease...so there's some rationale for thinking about trying to reduce chronic inflammation with something as simple as vitamin D. And it may have a further effect on atherosclerotic risk of cardiovascular disease."

In other words, lowering your cardiovascular risk and protecting yourself from just about every other chronic disease may be as simple as getting more vitamin D.

Unfortunately, as much as 80 percent of the U.S. population is vitamin D deficient.[13] And those statistics won't get any better any time soon as long as health "experts" in this country continue to push propaganda to avoid the sun completely.

The truth is, you can–and should–spend 20 minutes a day in the sun without sunscreen. This healthy exposure will help boost your vitamin D levels naturally.

Plus, ignore all the medical experts who continue to claim that taking vitamin D and measuring blood levels isn't important.

You should take a vitamin D supplement. Currently, the Institute of Medicine (IOM) recommends 600 international units (IU) of vitamin D daily for adults up to age 70. After age 71, the IOM recommends increasing intake to 800 IU. But these recommendations are based on findings regarding bone health.

Ongoing research proves you need much higher doses to achieve and maintain optimal vitamin D levels in the body. I recommend everyone take a daily, high-quality supplement that contains 5,000 IU of vitamin D. If you don't like taking too many pills or capsules, look for a vitamin D in liquid form. You can take it straight from the dropper or add it to any beverage you like.

CONQUERING EVERYDAY HEALTH

Part 5: The Insider's secret to conquering obesity

Chapter 26

Natural ways to soothe common digestive issues

Your digestive system is one of the most active parts of your body. But it's an often-ignored area of health. That is, until something goes wrong. And you get constipated. Or the opposite.

Maybe you've tried upping your fiber. You've tried a probiotic. Perhaps you've even given up dairy. But still no improvement. It could mean that your digestive system is missing three key nutrients.

Which ones?

Well, remember, the human body in an engineering marvel. So, let's think about this for a moment...

Your body must get certain essential vitamins from foods you eat. It can't make these vitamins on its own. So, when you eat food, what part of your body breaks down and begins to absorb these essential vitamins?

You got it–your digestive tract.

And these three key vitamins are *exactly* the ones that your digestive system needs. Unfortunately, very few of us get enough of these three essential vitamins from diet alone. So, what should work like a charm can turn into a vicious cycle when you don't get enough of these vitamins.

So, let's look at three main vitamins you need for a healthy digestive system:

1. **The B vitamins.** There are actually 8 B vitamins. And they are all essential for digestive health. But since they are water-soluble vitamins, you can't store them in fat cells or tissues. Therefore, you must get a regular supply from the foods you

eat. Or from a dietary supplement.

How do B vitamins aid digestion?

In general, they help move energy obtained from food into the tissue cells, where it is needed. In particular, vitamin **B1** (thiamine) helps convert carbs in the diet into energy. This fuels your cellular metabolism and helps regulate your appetite.

Vitamin B2 (riboflavin) helps keep the mucosal lining of your digestive tract in good shape. It also helps to break down proteins, fats and carbohydrates in the foods you eat. Without vitamin B2, you may have trouble digesting food. And converting the nutrients into energy. Low B2 can also cause tongue and mouth sores and swelling. Clearly, this uncomfortable situation will also interfere with normal eating and digestion.

Vitamin B3 (niacin) plays an important role in the breakdown of carbs, fats and *alcohol*. Lack of niacin causes pellagra, with severe vomiting and diarrhea. Obviously, this too will interfere with digestion and absorption of nutrients. And it can lead to dehydration.

Vitamin B6 (pyridoxine) helps the body process proteins in the diet.

Biotin helps produce healthy cholesterol. And remember, every cell in your body needs cholesterol. Biotin also processes proteins, carbs and fatty acids. And it helps eliminate the waste your body produces when it breaks down protein.

Folic acid is the final B vitamin related to healthy digestion. Research links higher levels of this vitamin with a lower risk of colon cancer. In addition, we know that low folic acid in women can result in birth defects. This is why many foods today, such as cereal and bread, are now fortified with folic acid.

You can find B vitamins in meat, dairy, eggs, green leafy vegetables, beans, seafood, and whole grains. However, studies show that many people don't get enough B vitamins from their diet. So, I recommend everyone take a high-quality B supplement.

2. **Vitamin C.** All the connective tissues in your digestive tract contain collagen. This protein helps hold your tissues together. Your body regularly replenishes this collagen to keep your tissues strong. And to heal damaged tissues in your digestive tract.

But you need vitamin C to make this all happen.

In fact, vitamin C helps your body produce enough collagen to keep the tissues of your digestive tract healthy. So, if you suffer from a bout of irritable bowels once in a while, make sure to take plenty of vitamin C to help your tissues recover.

Vitamin C is also important for healthy teeth and gums, a key to proper eating and digestion. Vitamin C also helps with healthy iron balance. (Most people do *not* require iron supplements. Getting plenty of vitamin C will help you get all the iron you need without supplements or fortified foods.)

Good natural dietary sources of vitamin C include berries, broccoli, citrus fruits, peppers, and tomatoes.

3. **Vitamin D.** Of course, many studies link low levels of the "sunshine" vitamin with a higher risk of colon cancer.[1] Indeed low vitamin D seems to increase your risk of many types of cancer. Deficiency also increases overall mortality.

But researchers are now beginning to look more closely at the importance of vitamin D in the colon, specifically. In fact, we now know that men and women who live farther away from the equator, in latitudes where the sun is weaker, get Irritable Bowel Diseases (IBD) much more commonly. Researchers think IBD, like multiple sclerosis, might have something to do with low vitamin D levels. Indeed, we already know that vitamin D plays a role in taming inflammation. And regulating the immune system. So it makes sense that Crohn's disease and ulcerative colitis, both inflammatory problems, might respond to vitamin D.

You find vitamin D naturally in foods like eggs, liver, and oily fish such as salmon and tuna. But about 1 billion men and women worldwide have a frank vitamin D deficiency. Including millions in the U.S. And up to 75 million having inadequate levels. So, I believe most people in the U.S. would benefit from a high-quality vitamin D supplement.

Of course, these three vitamins have many health benefits beyond keeping the digestive tract healthy. But as I said earlier, few of us can get to adequate levels from diet alone. So, I recommend finding high-quality supplements.

Drinking plenty of water is also essential when it comes to healthy digestion. Or better yet, drink *red bush* in your water. For 12 years I've focused a large part of my own research on a plant called red bush, or **rooibos**, native to South Africa. One of the most impressive effects of red bush is that it improves hydration all the way down to a cellular level. But I can also tell you about another benefit I've always heard about—both from doctors and South Africans who drink red bush: It also works wonders on digestion. Specifically, it helps digestive complaints such as indigestion and constipation. And red bush is safe. In fact, it's so safe mothers in South Africa give red bush tea to their infants because it helps with colic. From my experience, red bush is actually safe to drink instead of plain water—all day, every day.

These steps will help lay the foundation for overall healthy digestion. But you may need some additional support if you're suffering from a specific gastrointestinal disorder. Luckily, there are natural approaches that can help.

The drug-free way to put an end to irritable bowel

Inflammatory bowel disease (IBD) is becoming more commonly known each day. Which is good, because it can be a debilitating problem. So the more people know about it and talk about it, the more comfortable sufferers will be to seek help.

However, it's critical to choose the right kind of help. And it's not just people with diagnosed IBD (a.k.a. Crohn's disease and colitis) who need to be concerned about it. Irritable bowel syndrome (IBS), with related symptoms that afflict up to 15% of the U.S. population, may be a warning sign that IBD is coming for those who don't make a change.

IBS is a prime example of how the mind and body are connected. It's no surprise that the people who experience it and the chronic gastrointestinal pain or discomfort it involves often have a history of childhood trauma such as physical or sexual abuse, parental divorce, major illness or accident, or death of a loved one. It's the body's expression of the mind's suffering.

IBS also runs in families, so biomedical scientists are quick to claim some kind of genetic basis—but lifestyle factors run in families just as much as genes do.

How thin are your boundaries?

Tufts University professor Ernest Hartmann developed a "boundary concept" to explain differences in personality type. He found that people have differing levels of boundaries, ranging from thick to thin. Thin-boundary people tend to be more artistic, more connected with their dreams, and more likely to see themselves "merge" in their relationships with others. Thick- boundary people see clear divides between themselves and others and tend to see the world in black-and-white.

My colleague Michael A. Jawer and I suspected that this boundary concept could explain some mysteries of physical health, and we were right. In our book *Your Emotional Type*, we demonstrate that people with thin boundaries are more susceptible to a dozen illnesses with mind-body components—including IBS.

A common denominator among these ailments? Low serotonin levels. Serotonin is a key neurotransmitter found in the brain—but 95 percent is found in the neuroendocrine tissue of the gut. (Ever wonder why we have "gut feelings," and feel like we've been "punched in the gut" when we get bad news? It's likely related to these neurochemicals—chemicals that relate to thoughts and feelings—that are actually present in the gut.)

The level of serotonin in IBS patients (and, for that matter, fibromyalgia sufferers) is low compared with individuals experiencing the thick boundary condition of chronic fatigue syndrome. And while serotonin is far from the sole actor, the difference points toward a meaningful distinction in boundary type among these conditions.

Sufferers are often described as "overly anxious" and even "driven." It also often co-occurs with seasonal allergies and allergic eczema. And people with IBS are more likely to suffer from fibromyalgia and migraine. All thin boundary conditions.

A mind-body solution for a mind-body problem

If you have IBS, chances are you are a thin boundary type. (Find out your boundary type at www.drmicozzi. com.) Since the mind is clearly a critical part of what happens in this syndrome, your best bet for treating it is using a mind-body therapy that is most effective for your type.

Hypnosis is perfectly suited for people with thin boundaries. Biofeedback is another safe and effective technique for thin-boundary types. And acupuncture can be a powerhouse across the board—even for many people who have had no luck with other therapies.

When the syndrome becomes a disease

If IBS progress to an inflammatory bowel disease like Crohn's, treatment is a lifelong process. For many sufferers, conventional treatments offer little relief. Experts recommend complementary and alternative medicine (CAM) approaches, even beyond the mind-body disorder of IBS, as a powerful treatment for IBD.

My colleague, Joyce Frye, DO, who has contributed several chapters to my medical textbooks over the years and was previously with the Center for Integrative Medicine at the University of Maryland School of Medicine, was recently interviewed on this topic. "It's not a question of if you should use these alternative and complementary therapies," she emphasizes. "It's a question of using them correctly."

Another reason I urge you to find the CAM therapies that are proven to work for *you*—based on your individual type.

According to Dr. Frye, "The first goal is to treat the underlying imbalance that has caused a problem, so we can allow the body to heal itself. The second goal is to provide symptom relief in the meantime."

One of the best things about CAM therapies is that they are safe and unlikely to interfere with your conventional medical treatment. What's more, they can actually help you to replace essential vitamins and minerals your body is losing because of the disease.

Here's a closer look at some of the most effective mind-body remedies for bowel disorders.

Acupuncture

A recent review of studies on acupuncture and gastrointestinal diseases found acupuncture treatments to be helpful. One study in particular found that quality of life for Crohn's patients improved significantly after acupuncture treatments.

Mind/body techniques

Meditation, guided relaxation, yoga, and tai chi do not treat Crohn's disease directly, but they *do* reduce stress—and stress is known to trigger flare-ups and worsen symptoms. (If you choose the technique best suited to your emotional type, you may have even better luck.)

Hypnosis

According to a review by the University of Maryland Medical Center in Baltimore, hypnosis may help the functioning of the body's immune system and also give you the expected relaxation benefits of other mind/body practices, such as **easing stress and anxiety**.

Massage

Although it has no clear effect on Crohn's disease, massage is a popular stress reducer. If you experience the relaxation that comes from massage, ask your doctor for specific guidelines based on your medical condition, including whether the massage therapist should completely avoid your abdomen and how light or deep the massage should be.

Ginger, as well as verbena and linden teas may also help with digestion. In fact, I have some personal experience with the digestive benefits of these teas. They've been used in my family for at least five generations. But watch out for green and black teas which contain caffeine, tannins and oxalic acid—and can disrupt digestion.

Beware of this common peptic ulcer "cure"

Like other digestive disorders, peptic ulcers have frustrated mainstream doctors for decades. Their favorite 20th century approaches to medical problems—drugs and surgery—could not treat them. Much less cure them. In fact, you may have heard the old joke:

Nutritional help for digestive disorders

Dietary Fiber

Fiber, complex in any diet, is even more complex for people with Crohn's disease. Whether you should eat high-fiber foods or take fiber supplements depends on your specific condition and where you are at any given point in the disease. In some people, fiber supplements like psyllium powder (such as Metamucil) or methylcellulose (such as Citrucel) may stop mild diarrhea. On the other hand, if your Crohn's disease has caused adhesions and strictures, high-fiber foods will cause discomfort.

Probiotics

Probiotics are a type of beneficial bacteria that are found naturally inside our intestines and aid in digestion. According to Frye, "There is plausible rationale for why these would be helpful. If altered bacteria in the gut aren't the cause of the IBD, it certainly is an effect." I recommend getting probiotics from food sources such as yogurts or naturally fermented foods like sauerkraut or kimchee.

Omega-3 fatty acids are key nutrients found in fatty fish varieties, such as herring, salmon, bluefish, lake trout, and mackerel, and are available as supplements. Omega-3s have proven heart-health benefits, and they also have an anti-inflammatory effect, making them helpful in treating IBD. If you're going to supplement with fish oil, 1 to 2 grams is recommended.

Boswellia is an herb derived from the fragrant resin of a South Asian gum tree. In February I told you about its anti-inflammatory effects on joint and bone health. It's also commonly used to ease symptoms of IBD. A recent study confirmed that it can be

Continued on next page

effective in controlling inflammation caused by Crohn's disease and ulcerative colitis (400–500 mg/day).

Bromelain, an enzyme derived from pineapple, is a potent source of digestive enzymes. A recent study found evidence that bromelain might have beneficial effects in the gastro-intestinal tract for people with IBD. A good serving of fresh pineapple or pineapple juice will provide bromelain in a food matrix together with other nutrients.

Peppermint is Another effective digestion aid —which explains the ubiquitous "after-dinner" mints at restaurants. But instead of mint-flavored, sugar-filled candies, I recommend peppermint in the form of a dietary supplement or as a tea.

Ginger, as well as verbena and linden teas may also help with digestion. In fact, I have some personal experience with the digestive benefits of these teas. They've been used in my family for at least five generations. But watch out for green and black teas which contain caffeine, tannins and oxalic acid—and can disrupt digestion.

Q: *Who decides how to treat a peptic ulcer?*

A: *The doorman at the medical office building. If he points you to the internist's office, you get a drug. And if he points you to the surgeon's office, you get surgery.*

Truthfully, neither surgery nor drugs are good options for curing peptic ulcers. Both disrupt digestion, nutrition, and metabolism. And the drugs especially disrupt the absorption of critical B vitamins.

But about 20 years ago, many physicians thought we'd finally discovered the cause of peptic ulcers—a simple bacterium called *Heliobacter pylori* (H. pylori). They claimed we could "cure" the ulcer by killing the bacteria with antibiotics.

Proponents hailed this discovery as some great miracle. In fact, I knew a few of the simple-minded believers at the College of Physicians in Philadelphia, which I directed during the late 1990s.

A particularly delusional pair of doctors at the College had no patience for anyone who suggested that perhaps H. pylori was a normal part of the stomach's "microbiome." And they would never acknowledge that something else, such as stress, caused ulcers.

Instead, they could not wait to indoctrinate every physician with the new gospel. And they were disappointed when our program committee did not devote the entire year's continuing medical education program to this great discovery.

Well, somehow over the past two decades, they got someone to buy into this nonsense. In fact, they got a lot of people to buy into it. Today, many doctors give patients antibiotics in an attempt to eradicate H. pylori infections "causing" the ulcers. To add insult to injury, they give these patients proton pump inhibitors (PPIs) to reduce stomach acid while the stomach ulcer "heals."

But the healing never happens. Plus, you've wiped out normal H. pylori in the gut. And you've artificially lowered stomach acid with a drug. So now, when the patient goes off the PPI, the stomach acid comes back with a vengeance.

Plus, in a new study, Australian researchers found a strong connection between the eradication of H. pylori infections and rising obesity rates in the western world.

In their new analysis, the researchers looked at 49 studies with data from 10 European nations, Japan, the United States, and Australia. They found the higher the obesity rate in a population, the lower the rate of H. pylori infections. For example, research shows less than 50 percent of U.S. adults have the H. pylori bacteria in their gut. And we have one of the highest obesity rates in the world. Plus, in previous controlled trials, patients experienced significant weight gain after they eradicated their *H. pylori* infections with antibiotics.

These insights really aren't new.

We warned about it 20 years ago in Philadelphia. And Martin J. Blaser, M.D., Director of the Human Microbiome Program at New York University knew about it too.

In an interview, Dr. Blaser said, "In 1998, I predicted that doctors of the future will be giving H. pylori back to children. We should not be so fast in eradicating H. pylori."

It's just not nice to fool around with Mother Nature's plans, especially with antibiotics. These "magic bullets" are really "friendly fire." They cause more and more medical disorders and diseases.

Thankfully, more and more scientists like Dr. Blaser are now starting to realize the gut contains H. pylori for a reason. In fact, most people have H. pylori in their stomach. And most of them never get peptic ulcers!

In fact, we now know there's much more to the peptic ulcer story...

Peptic ulcers actually have a very strong mind-body connection. In fact, certain personality types (or emotional types) are more likely to develop them. And stress plays a major role.

Of course, my colleagues in Philadelphia never had any patience for the role of emotions in medicine. Except when it came to inflicting their own toxic brew of negative emotions on their colleagues and people like me whom they thought worked exclusively for them.

If you have a peptic ulcer, you should investigate ways to decrease your stress. Many mind-body approaches can help. You just need to figure out which approach works best for your personality type. For example, some people respond quite well to meditation. Others, not at all. Refer back to the techniques I outlined above for some additional suggestions,.

Of course, a good diet supports good digestion. And good

digestion nourishes the body. So do yourself a favor and start there. I'll tell you how in the next chapter.

Chapter 27

The Top of the Food Chain Cure for Obesity

There's a remarkable thing about nature: In all the various environments, or ecological niches, animals sort themselves out in a kind of "pyramid scheme"...with the biggest animal species at the top of the food chain.

In the ocean, the big fish eat the little fish, and the little fish eat the littler fish, and the littler fish eat...the plankton. But keep in mind that the biggest fish (actually a mammal returned to sea, probably related to the hippopotamus), the whale, actually feeds on plankton by straining tons of water through baleen (or whalebone) instead of teeth. How can tiny plankton cells feed the largest creature on the planet? The secret is volume and continuous feeding.

On land, the "top dogs," or the biggest animals at the top of the food chain pyramid, are fierce creatures like bears in North America and Europe, or lions in Africa, or tigers in India and Malaya.

One thing the bear knows...it's lonely at the top (of the food chain).

These animals, because of their large size, tend to eat alone and over relatively large areas... it takes a lot of food sources over a lot of territory to feed them. They are omnivores (eating everything) or carnivores (eating meat—the most concentrated source of food with plenty of essential fatty acids, bioavailable minerals and nutrients, calories and total nutrient density).

The exceptions to the solitary rule for animals at the top of the food chain are wolves and humans, who like to hunt and eat in groups (and as I pointed out in Chapter 24 of the previous section, there are some significant health benefits associated from this dietary "pack mentality.") However, while humans are like canines in eating together, we are like bears in eating everything, omnivorously.

A bit like the whale in the ocean, the bear feeds by taking in lots of little things—pounds and pounds of nuts, berries and other foods, including fish and meat when available in season. When some bears want to get their feet wet, they go jump in the river (in season) and are able to feed on salmon making their return runs to spawn—thereby getting plenty of meat, fats, and essential fatty acids (the omega-threes). But normally, the only way to get enough nuts, berries, and other foods to feed a bear is to cover a lot of territory and keep other bears and predators away.

And herein lies the secret…

The "top of the food chain" cure for obesity: Eating like a bear

After trying various fad diets that most young women fall victim to these days…my daughter Alicia decided to stop and take a cue from Nature. After taking a few advanced courses in biology she came to follow what she calls simply "The Bear Diet."

It was the healthiest and most effective diet she had ever tried for losing weight. And since it is also one of the most nutritionally sound diets I have ever come across, I endorse it wholeheartedly.

The Bear Diet includes plenty of nuts, berries, vegetables, fruits, and some meat when available. In addition to the high nutritional value of fruits, nuts, and vegetables, eating the bear diet requires "frequent, small feedings throughout the day"—like a bear. This provides plenty of bioavailable nutrients and essential fatty acids, leaving the you satisfied but thinner.

This diet also avoids health-sapping processed sugars and fats, and provides basically the same approach that works in controlling diabetes, heart disease, arthritis, and other chronic health concerns.

The proof is in the past—
our hunter-gatherer history

If you consider our prehistoric past, you'll find this approach makes perfect sense. Just don't get hung up on the misleading traditional picture of "Stone Age" humans that we've all been taught: "Man the Hunter." For the reality is actually closer to "Woman the Gatherer."

In fact, we have had the fortunate opportunity in modern times to observe actual human populations today that are essentially living in the "Stone Age" (*Neolithic*) in terms of the stone tools they use. Populations like the Tasaday of Mindanao, Philippines, the Bushmen of the Kalahari Desert, or even the traditional Inuit of the sub-Arctic. And in these "Stone Age" cultures, we observe that, mostly, it is the women who *gather* a lot of plants, nuts, berries, and small animals. And while the men may go away "hunting" large game, they mostly end up fooling around and getting into trouble.

A remarkable thing about wild game hunted and gathered is that the meat has only about 5% fat content—as opposed to the up to 50% fat content of artificially manipulated modern livestock raised for food. The USDA actually still considers that higher fat, "grade A" meat to be the better grades. But up until 100 years ago, cattle grazed on the western plains were still relatively lean—they had to be driven by cowboys (the original long-distance truckers) hundreds of miles to railheads for transport on trains to the stockyards in Chicago and elsewhere. Like the cowboys themselves, the cattle arrived pretty lean.

So while eating meat can be part of a healthy diet—watch out for what kind of meat. Natural, free-range livestock and wild game have the healthiest nutrient composition and are full of bioavailable minerals, vitamins, and other nutrients that are easy to digest and readily available to our metabolism. These lean, fresh meats will be free of the processed sugars and fats that are deadly causes of most modern ills.

And by the way, if anyone tries to tell you that humans should not eat meat...take a look at our teeth—do they look the teeth of a cow or horse?

On the vast American plains during the 19th century, Native Americans often suffered from what they called "rabbit hunger." During the depths of winter they could not hunt the declining populations of bison and other large game, instead, they had to rely on small game, like rabbits, which have very little body fat—and are very low in essential fatty acids. Contrary to some popular belief, not only is a little fat good for you, it is literally "essential" to health and life (that's why they are called *essential* fatty acids). Native Americans with "rabbit hunger" were starving from lack of essential fatty acids; when given just a spoonful of lard (rendered animal fat) they would return to normal health overnight.

In effect, getting the right amount of fat in the diet has always been a problem for people. Before the 20th century it was getting enough essential fatty acids, since they are rare in Nature, especially in plants. Today, we struggle from getting too much fat—and too many calories.

The Bear Diet provides just the proper balance. Plenty of bioavailable nutrients and essential fatty acids, which will leave you more satisfied...and thinner, too.

What to eat on the Bear Diet

Note that you do not have to count, measure, weigh, or otherwise obsess over what you eat down to the gram. This is a critical error that many of today's diet "gurus" and physicians make. Obsessive behavior around an activity of daily living, like eating, is not healthy and can be just another source of stress, which is counter-productive. When you follow the Bear Diet, how much you eat won't matter. And what and when you eat will easily become second nature.

1. Eat <u>all you want</u> (like the bear), of the following vegetables. (Eat them raw or cooked, without butter, fat, or salad dressing.*)

Artichoke

Asparagus

Bean sprouts

Beet greens

Broccoli

Cabbage (and pickled cabbage, or sauerkraut)

Cauliflower

Celery

Chinese cabbage (bok choy)

Cucumbers (and pickled cucumbers, sour or dill, not sweet)

Eggplant

Endive

Fennel (fenocchi)

Green beans

Endive

Escarole

Fiddle-head fern (in season)

Kale

Lettuce

Mushrooms

Mustard greens

Onions

Parsley

Peppers (red, green, yellow; hot or sweet)

Radishes

Rhubarb

Scallions

Spinach

String beans

Squash (green and yellow; zucchini)

Turnips

Watercress

Tomatoes

* A little olive oil with the vegetables is ok if you must. While not strictly on the bear diet, a little olive oil, while adding some calories, has other health benefits as demonstrated by the Mediterranean Diet. You can sautée with olive oil; or for fresh, raw vegetables, make a dressing of a little olive oil with vinegar, or with lemon.

2. Eat no more than 3 servings of fresh fruits each day.

Apple

Apricot

Berries (any kind; one-half cup = 1 fruit serving)

Cantaloupe (one-half medium-sized = one fruit serving)

Grapefruit (one-half medium-sized = one fruit serving)

Honeydew melon (two-inch wedge = one fruit serving)

Orange

Peach

Pear

Pineapple (one-half medium-sized = one fruit serving)

Plum

Tangerine or tangelo

3. Spices and seasonings (all you want)

Bouillon	Cinnamon
Herbs, including:	Cloves
Basil	Ginger
Chili	Mint
Dill	Nutmeg
Garlic	Horseradish, red or white
Rosemary	Lemon, lime
Sage	Mustard
Paprika	Tomato juice or paste
Pepper	(in cooking)
Tarragon	Vinegar
Thyme	

4. Eat several handfuls of mixed nuts (unsalted, not honey roasted). Especially almonds, pecans, and walnuts.

You can mix them with <u>small</u> amounts of dried fruits (careful, these can be high in sugar). You can have handfuls from a zip-lock bag throughout the day. This will definitely keep you from feeling hunger between meals. (Protein bars and "meal replacement" bars are not a substitute for anything. You will never need them and they should not form part of a healthy, weight loss diet.)

5. Once per day: Eat 4 to 6 ounces (about the size of the palm of your hand) of fresh grilled salmon or other fish, shellfish or seafood, squid (calamari; cuttlefish), or octopus (wild caught)

Grill fish with dill, natural yogurt, other fresh herbs, lemon-lime, cilantro, or onions to taste. Shellfish, while high in cholesterol, are low in fats. Eat mussels, clams, shrimp, lobster, or scallops cooked in their own broth, or sautéed in garlic and olive oil.

HOW to eat on the Bear Diet:

Start by completely eliminating carbohydrates from the diet for the first 2 to 3 weeks. No sugars, breads, starches; no corn, no potatoes, avoid "pulses" like beans (except green beans) and peas. This will help get your metabolism back on track and also provide some relatively rapid weight loss, which will be a source of motivation important to the psychology of dieting.

Start the day like a "hungry bear" coming out of hibernation. Try to start with the largest meal in the morning, since your metabolism will have all day to burn. However, if you are someone who just can't eat in the morning, then go with what your body is telling you. Don't eat when you aren't hungry.

On this diet, there is nothing magical about breakfast, lunch, or dinner. The cultural tradition of "three meals per day" is not a metabolic reality. You can actually "snack" throughout the day, like the bear, with frequent, small feedings.

You can eat the recommended foods in any order at any time. If you could not finish dinner (stop eating when you no longer feel hungry—it takes the brain a few minutes to catch up with the "satiety" of the stomach) have the left-overs the next morning.

After 2 to 3 weeks, and observing some real weight loss, slowly add back some carbohydrates in the morning, like a slice of whole grain bread, or a cup of steel-cut oats (not rolled oats), or even a bowl of Cheerio's (no- or low-sugar).

After another 2 to 3 weeks, as an occasional "treat," instead of snacking on the nuts and berries, you can have a small bag of pretzels, or other salty snacks, once in a while, but NOT sugary treats. You will find that nuts and berries take the place of all these sugary snacks and desserts.

Helpful Hint: Take a few minutes to prepare zip-lock bags and small containers the night before so you can accommodate your schedule during the day. By measuring out your snacks the night before, you will avoid "overdosing" on snacks.

Mix it up

A diverse diet is also important to gain a balance of different nutrients. Poor diets, and fad diets, that rely heavily on only one or few foods are inherently unhealthy and may lead to malnourishment. Europeans had a hard time achieving dietary diversity before their "discovery" of the Americas. There were only 16 different cultigens (plants cultivated for foods) in Europe from ancient Rome until the introduction of foods from the Americans in the 1600's. Tomato sauce did not appear on an Italian menu until late in the 1700's.

Of course, the bear may not typically eat all of these foods (like eggs and olive oil), but you can—and you will be very well nourished, keep your metabolism going, and experience healthy weight loss. When you achieve your desired weight there are many other foods and food preparations you can add back to your diet to maintain your health and your weight.

Chapter 28

10 tips for a balanced diet on a balanced budget

The mainstream media likes to lodge politically correct complaints that a healthy diet is too expensive for the average American. That's simply not true. Sure, if you only shop at overpriced places like Whole Foods and other upscale food emporia, you can blow your food budget. But those money pits are not the only places to buy high-quality foods. In fact, it seems to me that overpaying for food has become the latest fashion statement by urbanites, suburbanites, and the politically correct who aren't actually clued in to all the really important information about good nutrition.

Really, it's not rocket science. In fact, your grandparents knew just about all they needed to know about nutrition by living on the family farm. And there was nothing fancy about the family farm.

So, how can you watch your expenses while staying right at your usual grocery store? Well, the good news is, most regular supermarkets have already responded to consumer demand by supplying sections with fresh, healthy, organic foods of all varieties. Many also offer produce grown within 50 miles, so you can support local farmers instead of big agri-business.

With that in mind, here are 10 simple tips for improving your diet without breaking the bank.

1. **Forget all the fad foods.** As with too many dietary supplements, the current "it foods" are hot because of hype, not nutritional science.

   There is no reason to buy goji berries from the Himalayas at $14 a pound when raisins, for example, are filled with constituents like resveratrol, which have been *better* studied by science. And cleverly packaged pomegranate juice is good for you, but it's no better than any number of fruit juices in terms of antioxidants.

If you want to drink juice (though I prefer water—check out #10 on this list), you can approximate the taste of pomegranate juice—at far less cost. Just mix cranberry juice with a little lemon, both of which also have a host of health benefits.

2. **Choose your organics wisely.** Organically grown foods allow you to avoid pesticides and other agricultural chemicals. Organic makes sense with fruits and vegetables that you can and should eat with the skin: apples, celery, cherries, grapes, nectarines, peaches, pears, peppers, potatoes, raspberries, spinach, and strawberries. The skins have more vitamins. If a fruit or vegetable has a thick inedible skin, like bananas or pineapples, paying extra for organic doesn't make sense. When it comes to meat, milk, butter, and eggs, organic makes a world of difference in both healthfulness and taste. So it's worth the "splurge."

3. **Budget for beef.** Despite years of government health "experts" trying to convince the public that red meat will kill us, the fact is, red meat provides bioavailable protein, B vitamins, essential minerals, and a host of other nutrients hard to get from other sources. So forget everything you've heard from so-so-called government "experts," and indulge in a hearty steak—or bottom round, hanger, tri-tip, or shoulder cut. (Just make sure to budget a little more for the organic varieties. As I said above, this is one instance where it's worth it—from both health and taste perspectives—to spring for organic.)

4. **Don't buy bagged lettuce**. It may seem convenient, but bagged salad greens are ridiculously expensive and create unnecessary packaging and waste. Plus, the supposed convenience of not having to wash the lettuce disappears when you consider the fact that contamination appears to be more of a problem with bagged lettuce. Get your produce fresh, whole, and un-bagged. Another bonus: Un-bagged

produce stays fresh longer, since grocers water it periodically.

5. **Buy single ingredient spices in larger quantities.** Spices are herbal remedies by another name and they're calorie-free. So it's definitely worth budgeting for them. But make sure you're not paying more for packaging than for contents. Buy in bulk from natural food stores. Avoid expensive spice mixes and instead just use specific individual ingredients that are called for in recipes. Most spices will stay fresh for at least two years. (Powdered red spices, such as cayenne, chili, and paprika have a shelf-life of one year.)

6. **Make your own salad dressings.** There's simply no reason to buy bottled salad dressings. In addition to being expensive, they are full of unhealthy ingredients, fats, sugars and/or salt that have no place in a healthy salad. A basic— but delicious—salad dressing takes seconds to make. Just mix olive oil with vinegar or lemon oil. Then if you feel like it, throw in some of those healing (and calorie-free) spices for added flavor. To reap the health benefits of olive oil, choose a high- quality oil and keep it fresh by using it within three months. (By contrast, vinegar can be kept around for years.)

7. **Go nuts.** Nuts and seeds are loaded with heart-healthy essential fatty acids and other bioavailable nutrients and minerals, and they have been shown to lower the risk of many chronic diseases. They also help you feel fuller throughout the day, making them a good snack food. Although they're relatively expensive, a little goes a long way. Save by buying in bulk and keeping them in the freezer.

8. **Keep cereal simple.** Forget the pricey, high-calorie, pre-sweetened cereals, as well as the trendy (and spendy) designer granolas. Instead buy a big container of steel-cut oats. The only oats that are really heart-healthy are steel-cut, because they retain the healthy bran and not just the carbs.

   Use the oats to make old-fashioned hot oatmeal and add natural sweeteners such as maple syrup, honey, molasses, or agave. Toss in some dried fruit and nuts to make a quick, delicious, and inexpensive breakfast.

9. **Give your trash can a break.** Americans waste 15 to 30 percent of all the food they buy. When tomatoes get a little soft, chop them and cook them to make your own tomato sauce base. When vegetables begin to limp in the "crisper," use them to make your own vegetable stock. When bread turns hard, make breadcrumbs or croutons for your salads. When a recipe calls for egg whites, save and cook the yolk for a healthy sandwich or salad. When you buy a whole chicken, cook and consume the whole thing.

10. **Drink one thing.** There is no need to consume any type of expensive bottled beverages, carbonated sodas, or juice drinks. You are paying for bottling, transporting, and stocking drinks that are 99% water—a highly wasteful use of packaging, energy, fuel, and space just to provide products that "replace" water. Many of these beverages also contain unhealthy, high-fructose corn syrup or artificial sweeteners. Studies show that instead of being a healthier option, artificial, zero-calorie sweeteners can actually be just as unhealthy for metabolism, obesity, and diabetes as is sugar.

Instead, you should get the fluid you need from water. Of course, since today's public water sources are full of chlorine and toxic hydrocarbons, it's important to invest in a good filter. And to truly get the hydration you need—at the cellular level—I recommend adding South African red bush to your water.

Chapter 29

Your immune system's most powerful ally

It seems every time I sit back down to my computer, another study pops up about the importance of vitamin D. It's no surprise really - Vitamin D appears to benefit virtually every part of your body. And it seems to help protect you against nearly every chronic disease. Now, three new studies even illustrate vitamin D's incredible effect on the immune system.

In the first study, researchers looked at vitamin D and its effect on colon cancer risk.[2] They matched 318 people with colon cancer against a control group of 624 men and women without colon cancer. All the participants had given blood samples in the 1990s, before the appearance of any cancer.

The researchers measured the vitamin D levels in these samples and found the higher the participants' vitamin D blood levels at the outset, the less likely they were to develop colorectal tumors. Vitamin D, the authors suggest, interacts with the immune system to prevent the growth of this type of malignancy.

In a second study, researchers found that vitamin D prolongs survival time in people with metastasized colon cancer (cases in which the cancer has spread beyond the original site in the body).[3]

For this study, researchers followed 1,430 people with metastatic colon cancer. The patients in the lowest fifth for vitamin D levels survived for an average of 25 months. By comparison, patients in the highest fifth for vitamin D levels survived for an average of 33 months. That's 33 percent longer. In addition, higher vitamin D delayed any progression of the cancer from 10 to 12 months.

These findings make perfect sense.

You see, malignant tumors contain other types of cells besides the actual cancer cells, including T-lymphocytes or T-cells. These immune cells influence how fast a tumor grows or spreads. They attack cancer cells, which they consider "foreign," and can limit tumor growth. And research has shown that vitamin D is necessary to activate these T-cells.

In yet another recent study, researchers linked low vitamin D with poorer recovery after major surgery. For this study, researchers at Massachusetts General Hospital and Harvard Medical School measured vitamin D levels of patients admitted to the hospital's surgical intensive care unit (ICU). They found that ICU patients with low vitamin D blood levels spent more time on artificial respiratory support. Evidence links mechanical ventilation itself with a number of negative health outcomes. So getting off those breathing machines is a critical goal in critical care–and vitamin D helps.

Of course, we already knew that low vitamin D aggravates asthma and Chronic Obstructive Pulmonary Disease (COPD). Conversely, we know that boosting vitamin D levels improves lung function.

So a lot may come back to vitamin D's role in supporting immune system function. It appears this critical nutrient inhibits inflammation in the lungs, while boosting the immune system to defend against respiratory bacteria and viruses. Indeed, a balanced immune system *decreases* unhealthy inflammation, while *increasing* healthy immune response against microbes.

No simple-minded, single-function drug can do anything like that. All they do is put the system out of balance. They either boost the immune system artificially, which increases inflammation. Or they deaden it, which reduces inflammation, but leaves you vulnerable to infection (as with steroids).

It's remarkable that vitamin D positively influences the body's reaction to so many diseases–from cancer to lung diseases. And that something as simple as keeping up your vitamin D levels (as with daily supplementation) can translate into measurable and meaningful benefits–well beyond the high-cost, high-tech, and invasive modern medicine that we throw at these devastating diseases.

Unfortunately, the government-industrial-medical guidelines for vitamin D are so pathetically constrained by their focus only on bone health, just following the RDA for vitamin D simply won't provide the benefits this nutrient is capable of conferring.

You really need to take 5,000 IU of vitamin D daily. Even better, combine it with the natural powerhouse astaxanthin. You can now take them together as an easy-to-use and easy-to-absorb liquid.

P.S. A quick reminder: If you come down with the flu, you can safely take up to 20,000 IU of vitamin D per day just for the duration of the illness. This course will help your immune system fight the infection more effectively. And it will undoubtedly be a whole lot more effective than relying on the pathetic flu vaccine or Tamiflu drug treatment.

Chapter 30

10 signs you may have low vitamin D

I recommend having your vitamin D levels checked every 12 months through a routine blood test. Your doctor will order the test during your annual check-up. But between visits, and especially at the end of a long, dark winter, you should keep an eye out for 10 signs you may have a vitamin D deficiency.

An incredible amount of scientific evidence supports the need for higher levels of many nutrients for optimal health, including vitamin D.

Actually, the case with vitamin D is even a little different.

You see, with vitamin D, we are not just talking about how higher levels can prevent many common cancers, increase survival time, and improve quality of life in cancer patients. We're not just talking about how higher levels can help prevent heart disease, kidney disease, neurological diseases like multiple sclerosis, and other common problems.

There is, in fact, an actual worldwide deficiency of vitamin D. And evidence links many medical problems with this deficiency.

But government health experts wear blinders when it comes to vitamin D. They still only focus its role in bone health, which is based on discoveries made in the 1920s.

But in the last century, science proved that vitamin D is critical to every cell, tissue and organ in the body–not just the bones.

Medically speaking, there are 10 clear warning signs that you may have a vitamin D deficiency. Doctors see these signs every single day.

1. **Bone pain**

If you suffer from ongoing bone pain not explained by a "pathologic" diagnosis, you may have low vitamin D.

2. **Muscle weakness**

Muscles have vitamin D receptors and must have a constant supply to function.

3. **Chronic infections and respiratory illnesses**

Scientific studies show that vitamin D helps defend against infections and respiratory illnesses, especially in children. In fact, chronic respiratory infections in children are a strong indicator of a vitamin D deficiency. Instead of addressing this issue, the Centers for Disease Control wants all children to get the flu vaccine, which does not prevent the flu and appears to cause a six-fold increase in the risk of respiratory illness.

Thankfully, some doctors are getting the message. In fact, doctors with the prestigious Mayo Clinic advise that you need vitamin D to help your body fight infections. And if you're troubled by frequent infections, they advise getting a vitamin D blood measurement at your doctor's office.

4. Low mood

We know vitamin D helps produce adequate levels of serotonin, a critical neurotransmitter in the brain that produces feelings of well-being. And many solid, independent studies link low vitamin D levels with depression.

Of course, the popular "antidepressant" drugs on the market artificially raise serotonin levels through the roundabout way of preventing its re-uptake from the synapses. Unfortunately, these selective serotonin reuptake inhibitors (SSRIs) only work in one out seven patients. And new research suggests the one patient who *does* feel better after taking the SSRI probably *only* does so because of a placebo effect. Not because the drug actually works. Plus, SSRIs cause a wide range of harmful side effects.

Evidence links low vitamin D with increased anxiety, which frequently accompanies depression. Aside from clinical conditions like anxiety or depression, vitamin D's effect on serotonin can impact mood in anybody. So if your mood is off, it may be a sign of vitamin D deficiency.

5. Abnormal sweating

Abnormal sweating can be a sign of vitamin D deficiency. In fact, years ago, doctors commonly asked pregnant mothers if they experienced heavy sweating, since nutritional deficiency can occur under the strenuous demands of a growing baby.

6. Congestive heart failure

Maintaining sufficient vitamin D is a long-term, lifetime proposition. And if you don't maintain adequate levels over your lifetime, it even affects your heart muscle. In fact, the National Institutes of Health now recognizes scientific studies that show vitamin D deficiency can lead to congestive heart failure.

7. High blood pressure

Researchers link high blood pressure, a major cause of heart disease, with low vitamin D. In fact, a prospective study on women conducted by Harvard University over many years found that women with low vitamin D had 66 percent higher risk of high blood pressure compared to women with the highest levels of D.

8. Chronic pain

Studies show low vitamin D levels increase the risk of suffering from chronic pain. In fact, general malaise or fatigue may also be associated with lack of vitamin D. In athletes, lack of endurance may be a sign of low vitamin D levels.

9. Skin conditions

Your skin improves with moderate sun exposure. And studies show you can improve a variety of common skin conditions–such as dermatitis and eczema–by supplementing with vitamin D. In fact, many forward-thinking doctors now use vitamin D therapy to treat psoriasis patients. Plus, according to the Mayo Clinic, no matter what treatment is used, psoriasis is harder to manage unless vitamin D levels are adequate.

10. Kidney problems

Vitamin D is also important for the kidneys, which help make the active form of vitamin D in the body. So if you have kidney disease caused by cardiovascular disease or diabetes, low vitamin D contributes to this vicious cycle.

Simply getting older can make it harder for you to get enough vitamin D. The body just doesn't activate as much of it as you age. Of course, most the medical conditions I mentioned above also become more common with age. So while vitamin D is important throughout your life, it's especially important as you get older. Which is why it's critical to stay vigilant. Be on the lookout for any of the telltale symptoms listed above. And again, have your levels checked annually. The ideal vitamin D level for optimal health is 30 ng/ml or more.

To reach and maintain this optimal level, make sure to supplement with 5,000 IU of vitamin D daily. If you don't like taking pills, you can get vitamin D in a liquid form, which is now available together with astaxanthin, which you can take straight on the tongue or add to a small glass of natural fruit juice or milk in the morning.

SOURCES:

Part 1: Cancer Answers from a true insider

1 http://www.angio.org

2 Cavallo T, Sade R, Folkman J, Cotran RS (1972) Tumor angiogenesis: Rapid induction of endothelial mitoses demonstrated by autoradiography. J Cell Biol 54:408–420

3 Folkman J, Klagsbrun M (1987) Angiogenic factors. Science 235:442–447

4 Ausprunk DH, Falterman K, Folkman J (1978) The sequence of events in the regression of corneal capillaries. Lab Invest 38:284–294

5 Nature (impact factor: 36.28). 01/2006; 438(7070):932-6. DOI:10.1038/nature04478

6 http://www.angio.org/understanding/fact.php

7 http://www.scienceofcancers.org/brain-cancer-clinical-trials.php

8 "Vitamin C and Cancer," in *Nutrition and Cancer Prevention: Investigating the Role of Micronutrients.* New York: Marcel Dekker, 1989

9 "How Vitamin C Stops Cancer." *ScienceDaily,* 9/10/07. (Retrieved 5/29/12, from http://www.sciencedaily.com/releases/2007/09/070910132848.htm)

10 "Effect of vitamin C on prostate cancer cells in vitro: Effect on cell number, viability, and DNA synthesis," *The Prostate* 1997; 32(3): 188-195

11 Cancer *Epidemiol Biomarkers Prev* 1992; 1: 119

12 "Can dietary beta-carotene materially reduce human cancer?" *Nature* 1981; 290: 201-208

13 "Carotenoid analyses of foods associated with a lower risk for cancer," *Journal of the National Cancer Institute* 1990; 82: 285-292.

14 Omenn, G. S. (1998). "Chemoprevention of lung cancer: The rise and demise of beta-carotene," *Annual Review of Public Health* 1998; 19: 73–99

15 "Vitamins for Chronic Disease Prevention: Scientific Review and Clinical Applications." *Journal of the American Medical Association* 2002; 287(23): 3,116-3,129.

16 "Phase I clinical trial to evaluate the safety, tolerability, and pharmacokinetics of high-dose intravenous ascorbic acid in patients with advanced cancer." *Cancer Chemother Pharmacol.* 2013; 72(1): 139-146

17 "Phase I Evaluation of Intravenous Ascorbic Acid in Combination with Gemcitabine and Erlotinib in Patients with Metastatic Pancreatic Cancer," *PloS One* 2012; 7(1): e29794

[18] "Anti-angiogenic effect of high doses of ascorbic acid," *J Transl Med.* 2008; 6: 50

[19] Complementary and Integrative Medicine in Cancer Care and Prevention. New York: Springer, 2007, pg. 188-193

[20] www.californiaavocado.com

[21] Aggarwal BB, Bhardwaj A, Aggarwal RS, Seeram NP, Shishodia S, Takada Y. Role of resveratrol in prevention and therapy of cancer: preclinical and clinical studies. *Anticancer Res.* 2004 Sep-Oct;24(5A):2783-840. http://www.ncbi.nlm.nih.gov/pubmed/15517885?dopt=Abstract

[22] E. Brakenhielm, R. Cao, Y. Cao. FASEB J., 15, 1798–1800 (2001).

[23] K. Igura, T. Ohta, Y. Kuroda, K. Kaji. Cancer Lett., 171, 11–16 (2001).

[24] *In Vivo.* 2007 Mar-Apr;21(2):365-70

[25] *Journal of Experimental & Clinical Cancer Research* 2009; 28:124

[26] *Drug News Perspect* 2009; 22(5): 247-254

[27] *Molecular Cancer* 2011, 10:12

[28] Bhat TA, Nambiar D, Pal A, Agarwal R, Singh RP. Fisetin inhibits various attributes of angiogenesis in vitro and in vivo—implications for angio-prevention. *Carcinogenesis.* 2012 Feb;33(2):385-93. doi: 10.1093/carcin/bgr282. Epub 2011 Dec 1

[29] "Piperine inhibits PMA-induced cyclooxygenase-2 expression through downregulating NF-kB, C/EBP and AP-1 signaling pathways in murine macrophages," Food Chem Toxicol 2012; 50(7): 2,342-2,348

[30] "Piperine inhibits cytokine production by human peripheral blood mononuclear cells," *Genet Mol Res.* 2012; 11(1): 617-627

[31] "Piperine suppresses tumor growth and metastasis in vitro and in vivo in a 4T1 murine breast cancer model," *Acta Pharmacol Sin* 2012; 33(4): 523-530

[32] Crowley 1994:92; Lebot, Merlin and Lindstrom 1992:51-3

[33] Henderson B.E., Kolonel L.N., Dworshy R., Kerford D., Mori E., Sing K and Thevenot H. Cancer incidence in the islands of the Pacific. Nat. Cancer Inst. Monogr. 1985;69:3-81.

[34] Le Marchand L., Hankin J., Bach F., Kolonel L., Wilkens L., Stacewicz-Sapuntzakis M., Bowen P., Beecher G., Laudon F., Baque P., Daniel R., Seruvatu L., Henderson B. An ecological study of diet and lung cancer in the South Pacific. Int. J. Cancer 1995;63:18-23.

[35] Thevenot H., Germain R., Chaubet M. Cancer occurrences in developing countries. IARC Scientific Publication No. 75, Lyon, International Agency for Research on Cancer, 1986;323-329.

[36] http://www.steinerlabs.com/publications/alpha-pyrone-research-on-cancer-incidence/

[37] Castleman, Michael. "Kava Safety Update." *Mother Earth Living*; January, 2008

[38] http://news.uci.edu/features/can-kava-cure-cancer

[39] Mol Cancer. 2013; 12: 55. Published online 2013 Jun 10.

[40] Nutrition and cancer 06/2012; 64(6):838-46. DOI PubMed

[41] Kava Blocks 4-(Methylnitrosamino)-1-(3-pyridyl)-1-Butanone–Induced Lung Tumorigenesis in Association with Reducing O6-methylguanine DNA Adduct in A/J Mice. *Cancer Prevention Research*; January, 2014

[42] "Chemotherapy-induced neurotoxicity: the value of neuroprotective strategies." *Neth J Med*. 2012; 70(1): 18-25

[43] "Metabolic approach to the enhancement of antitumor effect of chemotherapy: a key role of acetyl-L-carnitine," *Clin Cancer Res* 2010; 16(15): 3,944-3,953

[44] "Induction of ER Stress-Mediated Apoptosis by a-Lipoic Acid in A549 Cell Lines," Korean J Thorac Cardiovasc Surg 2012; 45(1): 1-10

[45] "Lipoic acid - biological activity and therapeutic potential," Pharmacol Rep 2011; 63(4): 849-858

[46] "Coenzyme Q10 for Prevention of Anthracycline-Induced Cardiotoxicity," *Integr Cancer Ther* 2005; 4(2): 110-130

[47] "Improved survival in patients with end-stage cancer treated with coenzyme Q(10) and other antioxidants: a pilot study," *J Int Med Res* 2009; 37(6): 1,961-1,971

[48] "Vitamin C and Cancer," in *Nutrition and Cancer Prevention: Investigating the Role of Micronutrients*. New York: Marcel Dekker, 1989

[49] *Complementary and Integrative Medicine in Cancer Care and Prevention.* New York: Springer, 2007, pg. 178-186

[50] "Ascorbic acid and cancer: A review," *Cancer Research* 1979; 39: 663

[51] "A Prospective Study on Folate, B12, and Pyridoxal 5'-Phosphate (B6) and Breast Cancer,"*Cancer Epidemiology Biomarkers & Prevention* 1999; 8(3): 209–217

[52] "Multivitamin Use, Folate, and Colon Cancer in Women in the Nurses' Health Study,"*Annals of Internal Medicine* 1998; 129(7): 517-524

[53] *Complementary and Integrative Medicine in Cancer Care and Prevention.* New York: Springer, 2007, pg. 187-188

[54] "Calcium Supplements for the Prevention of Colorectal Adenomas," *New England Journal of Medicine* 1999; 340: 101–107

[55] *Complementary and Integrative Medicine in Cancer Care and Prevention.* New York: Springer, 2007, pg. 269-270

[56] *ibid*

[57] Mian L, et al. Review: The Impacts of Circulating 25-Hydroxyvitamin D Levels on Cancer Patient Outcomes: A Systematic Review and Meta-Analysis. DOI: http://dx.doi.org/10.1210/jc.2013-4320

[58] "Curcumin and its analogues: Potential anticancer agents," *Medicinal Research Reviews* 2009; 30(5): 818-860

[59] "Curcumin inhibits the migration and invasion of human A549 lung cancer cells through the inhibition of matrix metalloproteinase-2 and -9 and Vascular Endothelial Growth Factor (VEGF)," *Cancer Letters* 2009; 285(2): 127-133

[60] "Effects of curcumin on bladder cancer cells and development of urothelial tumors in a rat bladder carcinogenesis model," *Cancer* Lett 2008; 264(2): 299-308

[61] "Effect of curcumin on lung resistance-related protein (LRP) in retinoblastoma cells," *Curr Eye Res* 2009; 34(10): 845-851

[62] "Allicin inhibits cell growth and induces apoptosis in U87MG human glioblastoma cells through an ERK-dependent pathway," Oncol Rep. 2012; 28(1): 41-48

[63] "Allium vegetables and risk of prostate cancer: a population-based study," *J Natl Cancer Ins*t 2002; 94(21): 1,648-1,651

[64] "Inhibition of the Growth of Human Pancreatic Cancer Cells by the Arginine Antimetabolite L-Canavanine," *Cancer Res* 1994; 54(23); 6,045-6,048

[65] "GABA's control of stem and cancer cell proliferation in adult neural and peripheral niches," Physiology 2009; 24: 171-185

[66] "African herbal medicines in the treatment of HIV: *Hypoxis* and *Sutherlandia*. An overview of evidence and pharmacology," *Nutrition Journal* 2005; 4: 19

[67] "Medicinal plant 'fights' AIDS," BBC News, 11/30/01. (Retrieved 6/1/12, from http://news.bbc.co.uk/2/hi/africa/1683259.stm)

[68] "Anthropological study of health beliefs, behaviors and outcomes. Traditional folk medicine and ethnopharmacology." *Human Organization* 1983; 42(4): 351-353

[69] "Chrysanthemum indicum L. Extract Induces Apoptosis through Suppression of Constitutive STAT3 Activation in Human Prostate Cancer DU145 Cells," Phytother Res. 2012 (published online Mar 22)

[70] "Anti-inflammatory effects of the Nigella sativa seed extract, thymoquinone, in pancreatic cancer cells," HPB 2009; 11(5): 373-381

[71] Vitamin D deficiency and mortality risk in the general population: a meta-analysis of prospective cohort studies. *Am J Clin Nutr.* 2013(97):782-793

[72] American Cancer Society. What are the key statistics about

cervical cancer?http://www.cancer.org/cancer/cervicalcancer/detailedguide/cervical-cancer-key-statistics. Updated April 11, 2013. Accessed October 16, 2013

[73] JAMA Intern Med. 2013;():1-9. doi:10.1001/jamainternmed.2013.2912

[74] http://www.reuters.com/article/2013/02/27/us-lung-cancer-idUSBRE91Q16F20130227

[75] Rosenthal, Elisabeth. "Let's (not) get physicals," *The New York Times, Sunday Review*, June 2, 2012.

[76] "Treating you better for less," *The New York Times, Sunday Review*, June 3, 2012, pg. 12.

[77] "Quantifying the Benefits and Harms of Screening Mammography," JAMA Intern Med (http://archinte.jamanetwork.com/article.aspx?articleid=1792915), December 30, 2013

[78] "Rethinking Screening for Breast Cancer and Prostate Cancer," JAMA 2009;302(15):1685-1692

[79] Institute of Medicine (US) and National Research Council (US) Committee on New Approaches to Early Detection and Diagnosis of Breast Cancer; Joy JE, Penhoet EE, Petitti DB, editors. Saving Women's Lives: Strategies for Improving Breast Cancer Detection and Diagnosis. Washington (DC): National Academies Press (US); 2005.8. "Saving Women's Lives: Strategies for Improving Breast Cancer Detection and Diagnosis," National Institutes of Health (www.ncbi.nlm.nih.gov) 2005

[80] "Cancer? Not!" Medscape (www.medscape.com); Aug 29, 2013

[81] "The $2.7 trillion medical bill: Colonoscopies explain why the U.S. leads the world in health expenditures," *The New York Times* (www.nytimes.com), 6/1/13

[82] "Can colorectal cancer be prevented?" The American Cancer Society (www.cancer.org), accessed 8/2/13

[83] "Comparative Effectiveness and Cost-effectiveness of Screening Colonoscopy vs. Sigmoidoscopy and Alternative Strategies," *Am J Gastroent* 2013 108(1):120-132 (http://www.medscape.com/viewarticle/779647_4)

[84] "Less is More: Not 'Going the Distance' and Why," *JNCI* 2011; 103(23): 1,726-1,728 (http://jnci.oxfordjournals.org/content/early/2011/11/09/jnci.djr446.full)

[85] "The $2.7 trillion medical bill: Colonoscopies explain why the U.S. leads the world in health expenditures," *The New York Times* (www.nytimes.com), 6/1/13

[86] "Study: Colonoscopies often come with costly, unnecessary sedation," CBS News (www.cbsnews.com), 3/20/12

[87] Utilization of Anesthesia Services During Outpatient Endoscopies and Colonoscopies and Associated Spending in 2003-2009," JAMA

2012; 307(11): 1,178-1,184 (http://jama.jamanetwork.com/article.aspx?articleid=1105089)

[88] "Reducing Mortality from Colorectal Cancer by Screening for Fecal Occult Blood," NEJM 1993; 328:1365-1371

[89] "Colorectal-Cancer Incidence and Mortality with Screening Flexible Sigmoidoscopy," NEJM 2012; 366:2345-2357

[90] "Once-only flexible sigmoidoscopy screening in prevention of colorectal cancer: a multicentre randomised controlled trial." Lancet 2010;375:1624-1633

[91] "Once-Only Sigmoidoscopy in Colorectal Cancer Screening: Follow-up Findings of the Italian Randomized Controlled Trial—SCORE," JNCI 2011; 103(17):1310-1322

Part 2: Healing pain instead of treating pain

[1] http://www.neurology.org/content/80/5/424.extract

[2] https://login.medscape.com/login/sso/getlogin?urlCache=aHR0cDovL3d3dy5tZWRzY2FwZS5jb20vdmlld2FydGljbGUvNzc4MTEw&ac=401

[3] http://www.ncbi.nlm.nih.gov/pubmed/22529203

[4] http://www.ncbi.nlm.nih.gov/pubmed/14752215

[5] The Lancet. "Paracetamol no better than placebo for lower back pain." ScienceDaily. ScienceDaily, 24 July 2014. <www.sciencedaily.com/releases/2014/07/140724094025.htm>

[6] "Food and Drug Administration. Assessment of Safety of Aspirin and Other Nonsteroidal Anti-Inflammatory Drugs (NSAIDs)." Available at: http://www.fda.gov/ohrms/dockets/ac/02/briefing/3882b2_02_mcneil-nsaid.htm. Accessed February 18, 2014

Part 3: Brain-healers from behind the curtain

[1] "Higher normal fasting plasma glucose is associated with hippocampal atrophy: The PATH Study,"Neurology 2012; 79:1,019-1,026

[2] "Impaired insulin and insulin-like growth factor expression and signaling mechanisms in Alzheimer's disease—is this type 3 diabetes?" J Alzheimers Dis 2005; 7(1): 63–80

[3] "Berberine: A potential multipotent natural product to combat Alzheimer's Disease," Molecules 2011; 16: 6,732-6,740

[4] "Oren-gedoku-to and its Constituents with Therapeutic Potential in Alzheimer's Disease Inhibit Indoleamine 2, 3-Dioxygenase Activity In Vitro," J Alzheimers Dis 2010; 22(1):257-66

[5] Molecular Basis of Inhibitory Activities of Berberine against Pathogenic

Enzymes in Alzheimer's Disease," *The Scientific World Journal* vol. 2012, Article ID 823201 (doi:10.1100/2012/823201)

6   Effect of Vitamin E and Memantine on Functional Decline in Alzheimer Disease – The TEAM-AD VA Cooperative Randomized Trial," JAMA. 2014; 311(1): 33-34

Part 4: Master your heart health

1   "Blood tests for heart disease." http://www.mayoclinic.org/diseases-conditions/heart-disease/in-depth/heart-disease/art-20049357. Accessed March 24, 2014.

2   "Moderate elevation of body iron level and increased risk of cancer occurrence and death." Int J Cancer. 1994 Feb 1;56(3):364-9.

3   Muller H, et al. The Serum LDL/HDL Cholesterol Ratio Is Influenced More Favorably by Exchanging Saturated with Unsaturated Fat Than by Reducing Saturated Fat in the Diet of Women. *J. Nutr. January* 1, 2003 vol. 133 no. 1 78-83.

4   Nichols AB, et al. Daily nutritional intake and serum lipid levels. The Tecumseh study.*Am J Clin Nutr.* 1976 Dec;29(12):1384-92.

5   Dreon DM, et al. Change in dietary saturated fat intake is correlated with change in mass of large low-density-lipoprotein particles in men. *Am J Clin Nutr.* May 1998 vol. 67 no. 5 828-836.

6   Siri-Tarino, PW. Meta-analysis of prospective cohort studies evaluating the association of saturated fat with cardiovascular disease. *Am J Clin Nutr.* January 2010 ajcn.27725

7   Lemos da Luz P, et al. High Ratio of Triglycerides to HDL-Cholesterol Predicts Extensive Coronary Disease. Clinics. Aug 2008; 63(4): 427–432

8   Sachdeva A, et al. Lipid levels in patients hospitalized with coronary artery disease: an analysis of 136,905 hospitalizations in Get With The Guidelines

9   Weverling-Rijnsburger AWE, et al. Total cholesterol and risk of mortality in the oldest old. *The Lancet.* Volume 350, Issue 9085, 18 October 1997, Pages 1119–1123

10 Neaton JD, et al. Serum Cholesterol Level and Mortality Findings for Men Screened in the Multiple Risk Factor Intervention Trial. *Arch Intern Med.*1992;152(7):1490-1500. doi:10.1001/archinte.1992.00400190110021

11 Lack of Vitamin D Linked to CVD Biomarkers, Inflammation," *Medscape* (www.medscape.com) 2/27/2014

12 "Vitamin D deficiency is associated with inflammation in older Irish adults," *J Clin Endocrinol Metab* 2014

13 "Demographic Differences and Trends of Vitamin D Insufficiency in the US Population, 1988-2004" *Arch Intern Med.* 2009;169(6):626-632

Part 5: Conquering everyday health

[1] "Vitamin D and gastrointestinal diseases: inflammatory bowel disease and colorectal cancer," *Therap Adv Gastroenterol.* 2011 January; 4(1): 49–62

[2] "Plasma 25-hydroxyvitamin D and colorectal cancer risk according to tumour immunity status," Gut; published online 1/15/2015

[3] Vitamin D status and survival of metastatic colorectal cancer patients: Results from CALGB/SWOG 80405," *J Clin Oncol* 2015; 33

About the Author

Marc S. Micozzi, M.D., Ph.D.

In his 35-year career, physician, medical anthropologist and epidemiologist Marc S. Micozzi M.D., Ph.D., has accomplished something no other physician has been able to achieve.

He thrust the STAGGERING PROOF of complementary alternative therapies in the faces of mainstream medicine AND DEMANDED THEY LISTEN. In fact, some of the world's most recognized natural research—on things like lycopene, lutein, brassica vegetables, and excess iron—would not even exist without his courage to stand up for true science.

His medical career is all but unrivaled—especially given his vast and unique mixture of experience within mainstream medicine and complementary and alternative medicine (CAM).

Dr. Micozzi was the founding editor-in-chief of the first U.S. journal in Complementary and Alternative Medicine and organized and edited the first U.S. textbook in the field, *Fundamentals of Complementary & Integrative Medicine* in 1996, continuously in print for 20 years, now it its 5th edition. He has published nearly 300 articles in medical literature and is the author or editor of over 40 books.

As the Senior Investigator for cancer prevention at the National Cancer Institute, Dr. Micozzi published the original research on diet, nutrition, and chronic disease. He continued this line of research as the Associate Director of the Armed Forces Institute of Pathology and Director of the National Museum of Health and Medicine.

He has served as the Executive Director of the College of Physicians of Philadelphia (the same city where he completed medical and graduate training at the University of Pennsylvania).

In recent years, Dr. Micozzi has served as the Founding Director of the Policy Institute for Integrative Medicine, working to educate policy makers, the health professions, and the general public about the opportunities for integrative medicine and the need for clean, clear science within our modern medical establishment.

As Editor of his monthly newsletter *Insiders' Cures*, Dr. Micozzi's message of *taking what's rightfully yours* is already changing the lives of people just like you…

"You're making a difference in so many lives,"
writes Dan from Scottsdale, AZ

Elaine Fisher wrote in to say…
"Dr. Micozzi, thank you so much for the TRUTH and the diligence."

And Marlene couldn't wait to tell Dr. Micozzi,
"I treasure all of your information. I look forward to your posts like a bear to honey. BLESS YOU."

Books

Dr. Micozzi has written or edited over 40 books, including (with Michael Jawer), *The Spiritual Anatomy of Emotion* and *Your Emotional Type: Key to the Therapies That Will Work for You*. He was the founding editor-in-chief of the first U.S. journal on the subject of CAM (in 1994), and he organized and edited the first U.S. textbook, *Fundamentals of Complementary & Alternative Medicine*, now going into it's fifth edition.

"*The Spiritual Anatomy* of Emotion presents a unique and arresting view of such topics as mind, body, memory, illness, perception, and emotion. The authors show us an altogether novel way of understanding who we are and what we're about. There's more to being human than we ever imagine, and this book is an excellent road map for anyone who wants to take that journey."

ERIC LESKOWITZ, M.D.,
Department of Psychiatry, Harvard Medical School

"*Your Emotional Type*, may be the Rosetta Stone we've been waiting for—a code for matching a particular therapy to a particular patient. Micozzi and Jawer... have found gold."

LARRY DOSSEY, M.D.
Author of *Healing Words: The Power and Prayer and the Practice of Medicine* and *The Power of Premonitions*

"By helping patients understand the connection between their personality type, their symptoms, and treatment choices, Jawer and Micozzi help patients become more informed consumers of alternative health care."

ILENE A. SERLIN,
Psychologist and Dance Movement Therapist

You can read more about all of Dr. Micozzi's titles and purchase them online at www.drmicozzi.com.